Angiotensin II
Receptor Antagonists
Current Perspectives

Angiotensin II Receptor Antagonists

Current Perspectives

SECOND EDITION

EDITED BY

GIUSEPPE MANCIA MD

PROFESSOR AND CHAIRMAN

DEPARTMENT OF MEDICINE

UNIVERSITY MILANO-BICOCCA

SAN GERADO HOSPITAL

MONZA, MILANO

ITALY

informa

healthcare

New York London

First edition published in 2000 by Martin Dunitz Ltd.

Second edition published in 2006 by Informa Healthcare, Telephone House, 69-77 Paul Street, London EC2A 4LQ, UK.

Simultaneously published in the USA by Informa Healthcare, 52 Vanderbilt Avenue, 7th Floor, New York, NY 10017, USA.

Informa Healthcare is a trading division of Informa UK Ltd. Registered Office: 37–41 Mortimer Street, London W1T 3JH, UK. Registered in England and Wales number 1072954.

A CIP record for this book is available from the British Library.

Library of Congress Cataloging-in-Publication Data available on application

ISBN-13: 9781841845791

Orders may be sent to: Informa Healthcare, Sheepen Place, Colchester, Essex CO3 3LP, UK
Telephone: +44 (0)20 7017 5540
Email: CSDhealthcarebooks@informa.com
Website: http://informahealthcarebooks.com/

For corporate sales please contact: CorporateBooksIHC@informa.com
For foreign rights please contact: RightsIHC@informa.com
For reprint permissions please contact: PermissionsIHC@informa.com

Printed and bound by CPI Group (UK) Ltd, Croydon, CR0 4YY
Transferred to Digital Print 2012

Contents

Contributors

Enrico Agabiti-Rosei MD
Department of Medical and Surgical Sciences
University of Brescia
Brescia
Italy

Hans R Brunner MD
Division of Clinical Pathophysiology
University Hospital
Lausanne
Switzerland

John GF Cleland MD
Department of Cardiology
University of Hull
Kingston-upon-Hull
UK

Alejandro de la Sierra MD
Hypertension Unit
Hospital Clínic
Barcelona
Spain

Gianna Fabbri MD
ANMCO Research Center
Florence
Italy

François Feihl MD
Division of Clinical Pathophysiology
University Hospital
Lausanne
Switzerland

Guido Grassi MD
Department of Clinical Medicine, Prevention
and Applied Biotechnologies
University of Milano-Bicocca
Milan
Italy

Heiko Funke-Kaiser MD
Center for Cardiovascular Research (CCR)
Institute of Pharmacology and Toxicology
Charité – Universitätsmedizin Berlin
Berlin
Germany

Sverre E Kjeldsen MD PhD FAHA
Chief Physician and Professor
Department of Cardiology
Ullevaal University Hospital
Oslo
Norway
and
Adjunct Professor
Division of Cardiovascular Medicine
University of Michigan
Ann Arbor
Michigan
USA

Theodore W Kurtz MD
Professor and Vice Chair
Department of Laboratory Medicine
University of California
San Francisco, California
USA

Huan Loh MBBS
Department of Cardiology
University of Hull
Kingston-upon-Hull
UK

Aldo P Maggioni MD
ANMCO Research Center
Florence
Italy

Giuseppe Mancia MD
Department of Clinical Medicine, Prevention
and Applied Biotechnologies
University of Milano-Bicocca
Milan
Italy

Maria Lorenza Muiesan MD
Department of Medical and Surgical Sciences
University of Brescia
Brescia
Italy

Damiano Rizzoni MD
Department of Medical and Surgical Sciences
University of Brescia
Brescia
Italy

Luis Miguel Ruilope MD
Hypertension Unit
Hospital 12 de Octubre
Madrid
Spain

Ulrike Muscha Steckelings MD
Center for Cardiovascular Research (CCR)
Charité – Universitätsmedizin Berlin
Berlin
Germany

Giuliano Tocci MD
Faculty of Medicine
University of Rome
Rome
Italy

Fosca Quarti Trevano MD
Department of Clinical Medicine, Prevention
and Applied Biotechnologies
University of Milano-Bicocca
Milan
Italy

Thomas Unger MD
Center for Cardiovascular Research (CCR)
Institute of Pharmacology and Toxicology
Charité – Universitätsmedizin Berlin
Berlin
Germany

Peter A van Zwieten MD
Academic Medical Centre
University of Amsterdam
Amsterdam
The Netherlands

Massimo Volpe MD
Professor of Cardiology
Faculty of Medicine
University La Sapienza of Rome
Rome
Italy

Bernard Waeber MD
Division of Clinical Pathophysiology
University Hospital
Lausanne
Switzerland

Preface

Following their introduction into the medical armamentarium, angiotensin II antagonists have progressively gained ground and are now essential therapeutic tools, which are used to treat a variety of diseases. In the world of evidence-based medicine, this has been made possible by the design, implementation and completion of a large number of important studies. These studies have shown that this group of drugs offer protection against conditions such as hypertension, heart failure, post-myocardial infarction, primary and secondary prevention of stroke and prevention or management of diabetes and its renal complications. An update on this large new body of information is the aim of this book, which follows 6 years after the first edition.

During this period pathophysiological and clinical research has enormously increased the body of evidence on the clinical use of these drugs. First, angiotensin II antagonists have been definitively shown to be effective hypertensive agents both when used alone and when used in combination with several other drugs. Second, it has been shown that the action of these drugs offers a large nephroprotective effect in diabetes, the appearance and progression of renal damage being effectively delayed by their long-term use. Third, angiotensin II antagonists oppose the harmful effects of angiotensin II may offer a special protection against the occurrence or the recurrence of cerebrovascular disease. All this has been accompanied by trial evidence indicating that these drugs are useful therapeutic tools in patients recovering from a myocardial infarction or those experiencing heart failure both in the absence or presence of ACE-inhibitors. Finally, angiotensin II antagonists have been shown to prevent or delay the appearance of diabetes as well as to oppose the progression and favour the regression of subclinical organ damage. This is a fundamental aspect of future preventive strategies, which aim to maintain patients at low risk rather than having to intervene when a high risk and thus partly irreversible condition has already occurred.

This second edition of the book on angiotensin II antagonists, just as the first, is written by worldwide renowned experts in the pathophysiological and clinical aspects of cardiovascular disease. I hope its readers will find the book interesting and that it meets its intended goal.

A special word of gratitude is due to our publisher, Alan Burgess and Catriona Dixon, Production Editor, for their valuable assistance, which made publication possible.

Giuseppe Mancia

Angiotensin II antagonists in acute and post-acute myocardial infarction

Gianna Fabbri and Aldo P Maggioni

1

The role of ACE-inhibitors

Drugs which interfere with the renin–angiotensin–aldosterone system (RAAS) such as angiotensin converting enzyme inhibitors (ACEIs) have been available to clinicians for more than 20 years. ACEIs have been shown to be effective in treating essential hypertension, renal disease, and left ventricular systolic dysfunction as well as in improving survival after acute myocardial infarction. The first study that showed the efficacy of the ACEI captopril in improving the survival of patients with post-myocardial infarction (MI) left ventricular systolic dysfunction was published in 1992.[1] After this study the value of ACEI in reducing mortality rates and major non-fatal cardiovascular events in patients with post-MI heart failure/reduced ventricular systolic function or both has been clearly established by other randomized clinical trials and their overview[2–4] (Figure 1.1). On the basis of this evidence, these drugs are now recommended in patients with MI complicated by left ventricular systolic dysfunction, heart failure, or both. A different approach of using ACEI in patients with acute MI was tested in the same period. Nearly 100 000 patients with MI were treated within the first 36 hours from the onset of symptoms with ACEI irrespective of the presence of left ventricular systolic dysfunction.[5–8] This early unselected approach was associated with a significant mortality reduction, namely in the first 7 days from the beginning of treatment.[9] Finally, the indication for ACEI was further broadened to treat patients at high cardiovascular risk.[10–12]

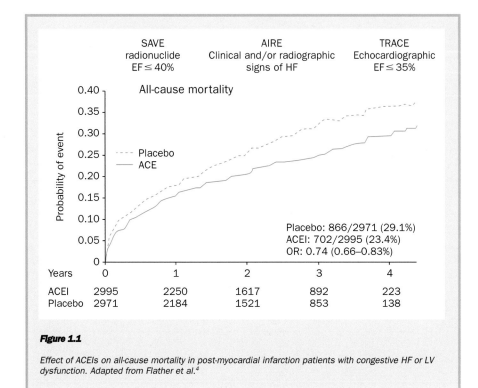

Figure 1.1

Effect of ACEIs on all-cause mortality in post-myocardial infarction patients with congestive HF or LV dysfunction. Adapted from Flather et al.[4]

A more specific approach: angiotensin receptor blockers

The inhibition of the renin–angiotensin system could have an alternative approach with the more recently developed angiotensin receptor blockers (ARBs). This class of drugs can offer a more complete blockade of the actions of the angiotensin II and improve the tolerability profile of this group of drugs. There are several reasons why an ARB might offer a more complete protection against angiotensin II and a better tolerability than an ACEI. Angiotensin II can be produced by ACE-independent pathways (chymase, kallikrein, cathepsin) and AT_1 receptor blockade would make more angiotensin II available to stimulate AT_2 receptors and perhaps other receptor subtypes. During treatment with ARBs there is a sharp increase in angiotensin II that works at the AT_2 receptors, producing vasodilation and inhibitory effects on cell growth. The blockade of AT_1 receptors at the same time as stimulation of the AT_2 has been shown to induce nitric oxide production and may increase generation of kinins at tissue sites. The elevation of the bradykinin levels with ACEI, even if it could contribute to the therapeutic benefits of ACEI, is associated with some of the adverse effects of these drugs such as cough, angioedema, and skin rash.[13]

The incontrovertible role of ACEI in heart failure and myocardial infarction has been a determinant in the evaluation of the effects of ARBs in these conditions: the need for direct comparison, including formally conducted tests for 'non inferiority' has implications in trial design, patient selection, choice of ACEI and dose, sample size, and end points.[14]

ARBs and myocardial infarction

ARBs in myocardial infarction have been evaluated according to the following approaches:

- head-to-head comparison with ACEI based upon the possible better tolerability of ARBs and the more specific and complete inhibition of the renin–angiotensin system (two trials)[15,16]
- add-on strategy (combination therapy) based upon the potential benefits of bradykinin and on the fact that, with the combination therapy, the rise in angiotensin II which occurs with ARBs (negative feedback) is reduced by ACEI (one trial).[16]

The OPTIMAAL trial was designed to test the hypothesis that losartan would be superior or non-inferior to captopril in decreasing all-cause mortality in high-risk patients after acute myocardial infarction. In this study 5477 patients with evidence of heart failure (HF) or left ventricular ejection fraction <35% were randomized a mean of 84.9 hours after the beginning of symptoms of MI to either losartan or captopril. The mean follow-up duration was 2.7 years. The trial selected the same dosage tested in heart failure in the ELITE II study: target dosage was 50 mg daily for losartan and 50 mg three times daily for captopril.[17] The study was event-driven and terminated after 946 deaths occurred. At the end of the follow-up period the rate of all-cause mortality was not significantly different in the two groups of patients (18.2% for losartan vs 16.4% for captopril; RR = 1.13, 95% CI = 0.99–1.28). No significant differences in the secondary and tertiary end point were shown. The secondary end point, sudden cardiac death or cardiac arrest, occurred in 8.7% of patients treated with losartan and in 7.4% of those treated with captopril (RR = 1.19, 95% CI = 0.98–1.43); fatal or non-fatal reinfarction rate was 14% vs 13.9% in losartan and captopril, respectively (RR = 1.03, 95% CI = 0.89–1.18). In the OPTIMAAL study the primary end point and all secondary end points showed a trend favoring captopril over losartan. Losartan was significantly better tolerated than captopril as shown by the rate of permanent discontinuations of drug: 17% vs 23% (hazard ratio (HR) = 0.70, 95% CI = 0.62–0.78). The conclusions of the authors were that in these patients, treatment with losartan conferred no further benefits in comparison with captopril. The findings of a trend toward superiority of captopril for all-cause mortality did not satisfy the trial's criteria for non-inferiority. For this reason, a possible superiority of placebo vs losartan could not be excluded.

Among potential explanations for the OPTIMAAL results, the most obvious possibility is that captopril is superior to the ARB losartan in patients with left ventricular (LV) systolic dysfunction or heart failure after MI. A second possibility is that the OPTIMAAL protocol was not optimal due to the type of population chosen or to the dose of losartan.

The first possibility is supported by the meta-analysis of Jong et al, which showed no difference in mortality for ARB vs placebo in patients with heart failure.[18] In this paper, 17 trials involving 12 469 patients with heart failure were included, the pooled outcomes were all-cause mortality and hospitalization for heart failure. There was only a trend in benefit of ARBs over placebo in reducing mortality (OR = 0.68, 95% CI = 0.38–1.22) and, when compared directly with ACEI, ARBs did not appear superior in reducing either mortality or hospitalization (OR = 1.09, 95% CI = 0.92–1.29 and OR = 0.95, 95% CI = 0.80–1.13, respectively). The effect of ARBs when compared with placebo (with or without background ACEI therapy) and ACEI in patients with heart failure has been analyzed in a recently published meta-analysis by Lee et al;[19] 24 trials involving 38 080 patients were included. The analysis revealed that ARBs treatment was associated with:

1. Reduced total mortality and HF hospitalization in comparison with placebo (OR = 0.83, 95% CI = 0.69–1.00 and OR = 0.64, 95% CI = 0.53–0.78, respectively).
2. No differences vs ACEI in all-cause mortality (OR = 1.06, 95% CI = 0.90–1.26) and HF hospitalization (OR = 0.95, 95% CI = 0.80–1.13).
3. Reduced HF hospitalization (OR = 0.77, 95% CI = 0.69–0.87), in a comparison of ARBs plus ACEI combination vs ACEI alone, without a significant reduction in total mortality (OR = 0.97, 95% CI = 0.87–1.08).

Because the comparison of ARBs versus placebo was, in this analysis, heavily influenced by the CHARM-Alternative,[20] the authors performed a sensitivity analysis by excluding data from that study: there was a non-statistically significant reduction in all-cause mortality (OR = 0.62, 95% CI = 0.36–1.07), whereas the HF hospitalization outcome remained significantly lower with ARBs (OR = 0.53, 95% CI = 0.30–0.97).

The most likely protocol-related explanation for the findings of OPTIMAAL is the choice of dose of losartan. The dose of captopril was well supported by the results of the SAVE study, whereas the dose of losartan was chosen with much less supporting data. The ELITE I trial[21] showed a superiority of 50 mg of losartan vs captopril in terms of mortality, but the trial was underpowered to test the effect of losartan on hard end points such as mortality. When an appropriately sized trial was planned (ELITE II), there was no evidence of superiority of losartan vs captopril, such as in OPTIMAAL. Different results were observed when a higher dosage of losartan was tested.

The results of the LIFE[22] and RENAAL studies[23] showed the beneficial effects of losartan when used at the dosage of 100 mg. In support of the hypothesis that the dose of OPTIMAAL could be inadequate are also the results of the IRMA study, which suggests that a dose response can exist with the ARB irbesartan in patients with diabetes, hypertension, and microalbuminuria. In this trial, 300 mg of irbesartan resulted in a superior renoprotective effect and in a trend toward a reduction of cardiovascular events as compared with 150 mg of irbesartan.[24] An adjunctive problem in the OPTIMAAL trial could have been the relatively slow uptitration of the study medication. Post-MI LV remodeling has two phases.[25-26] The first phase is the first 3–7 days after the infarction and consists of scar stretching: this process accounts for a significant proportion of long-term LV dilation and can be partially reversed by the early initiation of therapy with captopril.[27] The second phase, which progresses more slowly, consists of myocardial hypertrophy and ventricular shape distortion and can be effected by an ACEI at any time after MI. Many studies which included post-MI patients showed that ACEI exerted their beneficial effects on survival in the first week after MI.[28] In the OPTIMAAL study, patients were randomized an average of 84.9 hours after MI to either losartan 12.5 mg once a day or captopril 12.5 mg three times a day and uptitrated to 50 mg daily of losartan after an average of 8–9 days post-MI, long after the early phase of remodeling and the proven effects of ACEI and probably of ARB.

The VALIANT study investigated the effect of valsartan alone, captopril alone, or the combination of the two drugs. The population of the trial comprised patients with at least one of the characteristics necessary to be enrolled in the three reference studies AIRE, SAVE, and TRACE in which ACEI were shown to be effective in improving survival. Patients had to be enrolled between 12 hours and 10 days after the onset of symptoms of an acute MI and had to have evidence of LV systolic dysfunction (ejection fraction ≤40% at radionuclide ventriculography or ≤35% at echocardiography or an echo wall motion index ≤1.2 measured according to the method adopted by the TRACE investigators), and/or clinical evidence of heart failure.

The trial had been designed to enrol 14 500 patients. Being event-driven, 2700 deaths should be reached to provide a power of 86–95% to detect a reduction of 15–17.5% in all-cause mortality. In the case that valsartan emerged as non-superior to captopril, the study protocol planned to assess a non-inferiority hypothesis. On the basis of the reduction in mortality with the use of ACEI in previous trials (26% reduction in the overview of the three major trials SAVE, AIRE, TRACE), the threshold indicating the non-inferiority for valsartan was fixed at 1.13. This threshold allows us to preserve at least 55% of the survival benefit of an ACEI. Patients were enrolled and randomly assigned in a 1:1:1 ratio to the three treatment arms by 931 participating centers from 24 countries. Valsartan was started at the dosage of 40 mg bid, whereas captopril at the proven dosage of 25 mg tid. Doses were then gradually increased to their maximal dosage (valsartan alone, 160 mg bid; captopril alone or in combination, 50 mg tid; valsartan in combination, 80 mg bid) in four steps over 90 days. The primary end point of the study was all-cause mortality. The secondary end point was the combination of death from cardiovascular cause, recurrent myocardial infarction, or hospitalization for heart failure (Figure 1.2).

Over the median follow-up period of 24.7 months, the mortality rates in the valsartan, captopril, and combination groups were 19.9%, 19.5%, and 19.3%, respectively, showing, therefore, no significant differences among the three groups.[29]

The rate of the secondary composite end point (cardiovascular death, recurrent MI, heart failure) also did not differ significantly: 31.1%, 31.1%, and 31.9% in the three groups. In the

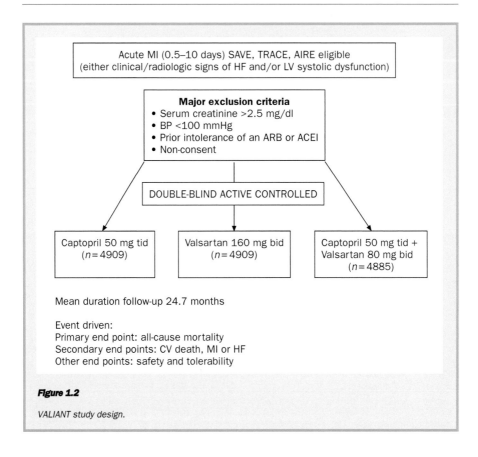

Figure 1.2

VALIANT study design.

non-inferiority analysis, the ARB valsartan was proven as good as captopril in reducing the risk of death in these patients, maintaining the 99.6% of the benefit of the proven dosage of the ACEI captopril (Figure 1.3). This finding was similar for the composite outcome and among subgroups of patients based on age, sex, previous medical conditions, and treatments.

All treatments were generally well tolerated. Patients taking both medications in combination, however, experienced a significantly greater number of drug-related adverse events. This group had the highest rate of treatment discontinuation (9%), whereas the lowest was that observed in the valsartan alone group (5.8%).

The pattern of adverse events differed between captopril (more cough, rash, and taste disturbance) and valsartan (more hypotension and renal abnormalities).

The favorable results of VALIANT raised the question of whether these results can be assumed as a 'class effect'. The differences in pharmacological profile among ARBs and the lack of direct

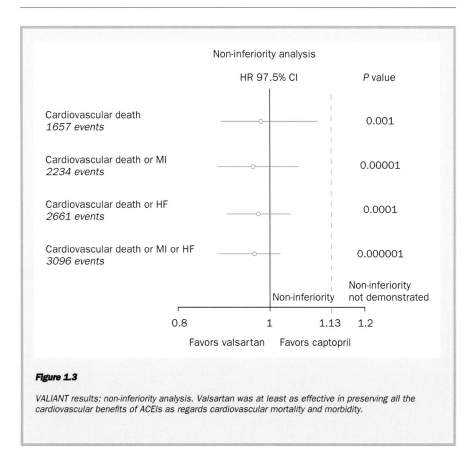

Figure 1.3

VALIANT results: non-inferiority analysis. Valsartan was at least as effective in preserving all the cardiovascular benefits of ACEIs as regards cardiovascular mortality and morbidity.

comparison trials in post-MI patients should lead us to be cautious. The editorial accompanying the VALIANT results says:

'Given that ACE-I have been shown to reduce the risk of death and non fatal cardiovascular events after acute myocardial infarction in 100,000 patients whereas the clinical experience with angiotensin receptor blockers has been more limited, and given that the cost of using valsartan at the doses used in VALIANT is approximately four to six times as high as the cost of using captopril, ACE-I remain the first-line therapy in high-risk patients with myocardial infarction. For those patients who cannot tolerate ACE-I, . . . there is a safe and equally alternative strategy . . ..'[30]

Therefore, even if a class effect cannot be excluded, the available evidence supports the use of valsartan in patients with post-MI LV dysfunction or heart failure or both because we have robust information on the effective dosage of the drug.

VALIANT is also the only study carried out in the post-MI setting that has reported survival in patients taking the combination of ARB and ACEI compared with those taking ACEI alone. The combination treatment was titrated to 80 mg twice daily for valsartan added to captopril 50 mg thrice daily. Mortality and the prespecified secondary outcome were not reduced by the combination of the two drugs compared with the proven dose of captopril, in front of a greater rate of adverse reactions. For this reason, the combination of the two classes of drugs is not recommended in post-MI patients complicated by LV systolic dysfunction/heart failure or both. These conclusions differ from those raised by trials testing ARBs in the setting of chronic heart failure.

ARBs and chronic heart failure

In the last few years, ARBs have been studied in many trials in patients with heart failure and LV dysfunction; in particular, the CHARM program and the Val-HeFT study have been completed.[31,32] In the CHARM-Alternative trial, candesartan was tested vs placebo in patients with reduced systolic function and heart failure who previously were found intolerant to ACEI. The results were similar to those achieved with ACEI in the past: overall mortality and HF hospitalizations were reduced by 23%. In the CHARM-Added trial, the combination of an ACEI with candesartan in patients with heart failure was tested. Such a combined therapy further reduced mortality and HF hospitalization by 15%, but its side effects were worse.[33]

Putting together the data from the CHARM-Alternative and CHARM-Added trials, candesartan treatment was found to be associated with a significant all-cause mortality reduction.

The CHARM results together with the Val-HeFT data, which showed a superiority of valsartan versus placebo in terms of morbidity and mortality, suggest that the combination of ARBs and ACEI in patients with chronic HF is beneficial in improving patient outcome. There are several possible explanations for this discrepancy between outcomes in HF and MI: clinical differences, time course and degree of RAAS activation, RAAS escape and dose of background ACEI treatment or of valsartan added. Patients with HF have a linear rate of adverse outcome, whereas in patients with MI the rate of events is higher in the first few months after the acute event. Moreover, patients with MI have a short-lived but acute neuroendocrine activation, with plasma concentrations of angiotensin II peaking after nearly 3 days, whereas HF is associated with long-term but modest activation of the RAAS. The tolerability of two inhibitors of RAAS in the unstable setting of MI could be less than for those in an HF setting.[34] In the CHARM-Added trial and in the Val-HeFT trial, therapy with ARBs was started in patients receiving long-term ACEI treatment. In these patients, an RAAS escape could have occurred with angiotensin II production by pathways other than ACE and the addition of an ARB can produce adjunctive beneficial effects. In MI patients enrolled in VALIANT, the RAAS escape did not occur and administration of just one blocker of the RAAS can be beneficial.

Finally, the dose of background ACEI may have a role in the different results obtained for HF and MI. The mean dosage of captopril in the combination arm of VALIANT was 107 mg compared with 80 mg in the two trials of heart failure.

The 1999 American College of Cardiology/American Heart Association (ACC/AHA) Guidelines for the management of patients with myocardial infarction did not mention ARB.[35] The 2001 ACC/AHA guidelines for evaluation and management of heart failure state:

> ARB should not be considered equivalent or superior to ACE-I in the treatment of heart failure and thus they should not be used for the treatment of heart failure in patients who have no prior use of an ACE-I and should not be substituted for ACE-I in patients who are tolerating ACE-I without difficulty.[36]

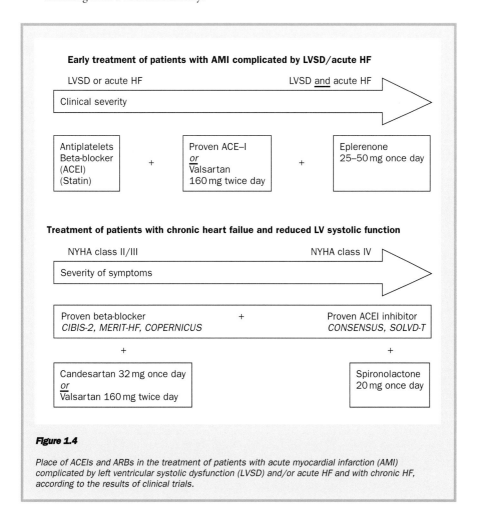

Figure 1.4

Place of ACEIs and ARBs in the treatment of patients with acute myocardial infarction (AMI) complicated by left ventricular systolic dysfunction (LVSD) and/or acute HF and with chronic HF, according to the results of clinical trials.

The 2004 ACC/AHA Guidelines for MI highlight that the use of ARB has not been explored as thoroughly as ACEI in patients with STEMI and given the[37,38] extensive randomized trial and routine clinical experience with ACEI they remain the logical first agent for inhibition of the RAAS. However, on the basis of these trial results, the prescription of an ARB is recommend at discharge to those ST-elevation infarction patients who are intolerant of an ACEI and have either clinical or radiological signs of heart failure and LV ejection fraction less than 40%.

Figure 1.4 summarizes the recommendations for the pharmacological treatment of patient with chronic HF and with post-MI LV systolic dysfunction/acute heart failure.

The decision in individual patients may be influenced by physician and patient preference, cost, and anticipated side-effect profile.

References

1. Pfeffer MA, Braunwald E, Moye LA et al. Effect of captopril on mortality and morbidity in patients with left ventricular dysfunction after myocardial infarction: results of the Survival and Ventricular Enlargement trial. N Engl J Med 1992; 327:669–77.
2. The Acute Infarction Ramipril Efficacy (AIRE) Study Investigators. Effect of ramipril on mortality and morbidity of survivors of acute myocardial infarction with clinical evidence of heart failure. Lancet 1993; 342:821–8.
3. Trandolapril Cardiac Evaluation (TRACE) Study Group. A clinical trial of the angiotensin converting enzyme inhibitor trandolapril in patients with left ventricular dysfunction after myocardial infarction. N Engl J Med 1995; 333:1670–6.
4. Flather MD, Yusuf S, Kober L et al. Long term ACE-inhibitor therapy in patients with heart failure or left ventricular dysfunction: a systematic overview of data from individual patients. ACE-Inhibitor Myocardial Infarction Collaborative Group. Lancet 2000; 355:1575–81.
5. Swedberg K, Held P, Kiekshus J et al. Effects of the early administration of enalapril on mortality in patients with acute myocardial infarction. Results of the Cooperative New Scandinavian Enalapril Survival Study II (CONSENSUS II). N Engl J Med 1992; 327:678–84.
6. GISSI-3: effects of lisinopril and transdermal glyceryl trinitrate singly and together on 6-week mortality and ventricular function after acute myocardial infarction. Gruppo Italiano per lo Studio della Sopravvivenza nell'infarto Miocardico. Lancet 1994; 343:1115–22.
7. ISIS-4: a randomized factorial trial assessing early oral captopril, oral mononitrate, and intravenous magnesium sulphate in 58,050 patients with suspected acute myocardial infarction. (Fourth International Study of Infarct Survival) Collaborative Group. Lancet 1995; 345:669–85.
8. CCS-1: oral captopril versus placebo among 14,962 patients with suspected acute myocardial infarction: a multicenter, randomized, double-blind, placebo controlled clinical trial. Chinese Cardiac Study (CCS-1) Collaborative Group. Chin Med J 1997; 110:834–8.
9. Ace Inhibitor Myocardial Infarction Collaborative Group. Indications for ACE inhibitors in the early treatment of acute myocardial infarction. Systematic overview of individual data from 100,000 patients in randomized trials. Circulation 1998; 97:2202–12.
10. The Heart Outcomes Prevention Evaluation Study Investigators (HOPE). Effects of angiotensin converting enzyme inhibitor, ramipril, on cardiovascular events in high risk patients. N Engl J Med 2000; 342:145–53.
11. The European trial On reduction of cardiac events with Perindopril in stable coronary Artery disease Investigators. Efficacy of perindopril in reduction of cardiovascular events among patients with stable coronary artery disease: randomized, double-blind, placebo-controlled, multicentre trial (the EUROPA study). Lancet 2003; 362:782–8.

12. The PEACE trial Investigators. Angiotensin-converting enzyme inhibition in stable coronary artery disease. N Engl J Med 2004; 351:2058–68.
13. Witherow FN, Helmy A, Webb DJ et al. Bradykinin contributes to the vasodilator effect of chronic angiotensin-converting enzyme inhibition in patients with heart failure. Circulation 2001; 104:2177–81.
14. Committee for Proprietary Medicinal Products. Points to consider on switching between superiority and non inferiority. Br J Clin Pharmacol 2001; 52:223–8.
15. Dickstein K, Kjeskshus J, OPTIMAAL Steering Committee of the OPTIMAAL Study Group. Effects of losartan and captopril on mortality and morbidity in high risk patients after acute myocardial infarction: the OPTIMAAL randomised trial. Optimal Trial in Myocardial Infarction with Angiotensin II Antagonist Losartan. Lancet 2002; 360:752–60.
16. Pfeffer MA, McMurray JJ, Leizorovicz A et al. VALsartan In Acute myocardial iNfarcTion trial (VALIANT): rationale and design. Am Heart J 2000; 140:727–34.
17. Pitt B, Poole-Wilson PA, Segal R et al. Effect of losartan compared with captopril on mortality in patients with symptomatic heart failure: randomised trial the Losartan Heart Failure Survival Study ELITE II. Lancet 2000; 355:1582–7.
18. Jong P, Demers C, McKelvie RS et al. Angiotensin receptor blockers in heart failure: meta-analysis of randomized controlled trials. J Am Coll Cardiol 2002; 39:463–70.
19. Lee VC, Rhew DC, Dylan M et al. Meta-analysis: angiotensin receptor blockers in chronic heart failure and high risk acute myocardial infarction. Ann Intern Med 2004; 141:693–704.
20. Granger CB, McMurray JJ, Yusuf S et al, for the CHARM Investigators and committees. Effect of candesartan in patients with chronic heart failure and reduced left ventricular systolic function intolerant to angiotensin converting enzyme inhibitors: the CHARM-Alternative trial. Lancet 2003; 326:772–6.
21. Pitt B, Segal R, Martinez FA et al. Randomized trial of losartan versus captopril in patients over 65 with heart failure (Evaluation of Losartan in the Elderly Study, ELITE). Lancet 1997; 347:747–52.
22. Dahlof B, Devereux RB, Kjeldsen SE et al. Cardiovascular morbidity and mortality in the Losartan Intervention For Endpoint reduction in hypertension study (LIFE): a randomized trial against atenolol. Lancet 2002; 359:995–1003.
23. Brenner BM, Cooper ME, de Zeeuw D et al. Effect of losartan on renal and cardiovascular outcomes in patients with type 2 diabetes and nephropathy. N Engl J Med 2001; 345:861–9.
24. Parving HH, Lehnert H, Brochner-Mortensen J et al. The effect of irbesartan on the development of diabetic nephropathy in patients with type 2 diabetes. N Eng J Med 2001; 345:870–8.
25. Jugdutt BI. Prevention of ventricular remodeling post myocardial infarction timing and duration of therapy. Can J Cardiol 1993; 9:103–14.
26. Pfeffer MA, Braunwald E. Ventricular remodelling after myocardial infarction. Experimental observations and clinical implications. Circulation 1990; 81:1161–72.
27. Sharpe N, Smith H, Murphy J et al. Early prevention of left ventricular systolic dysfunction after myocardial infarction with angiotensin converting enzyme inhibition. Lancet 1991; 337:872–6.
28. Latini R, Maggioni AP, Flather M et al. ACE inhibitor use in patients with myocardial infarction. Summary of the evidence from clinical trials. Circulation 1995; 92: 3132–7.
29. Pfeffer MA, McMurray JJV, Velazquez EJ et al. Valsartan, captopril or both in myocardial infarction complicated by heart failure, left ventricular dysfunction or both. N Engl J Med 2003; 349:1843–906.
30. Mann DL, Deswal A. Angiotensin receptor blockade in acute myocardial infarction – a matter of dose. N Engl J Med 2003; 349:1963–5.
31. Pfeffer MA, Swedberg K, Granger CB et al for the CHARM Investigators and committees. Effects of candesartan on mortality and morbidity in patients with chronic heart failure: the CHARM-Overall programme. Lancet 2003; 362:759–66.
32. Cohn JN, Tognoni G. Valsartan Heart Failure Trial Investigators. A randomized trial of the angiotensin-receptor blocker valsartan in chronic heart failure. N Engl J Med 2001; 345:1667–75.
33. McMurray JJ, Ostergren J, Swedberg K et al for the CHARM Investigators and committees. Effect of candesartan in patients with chronic heart failure and reduced left ventricular systolic function taking angiotensin converting enzyme inhibitors: the CHARM-Added trial. Lancet 2003; 362:767–71.
34. McAlpine HM, Morton JJ, Leckie B et al. Neuroendocrine activation after acute myocardial infarction. Br Heart J 1988; 60:117–24.

35. ACC/AHA Guidelines for the management of patients with acute myocardial infarction. Circulation 1999; 100:1016–30.

36. ACC/AHA Guidelines for the evaluation and management of chronic heart failure in the adult. J Am Coll Cardiol 2001; 38:2101–13.

37. ACC/AHA Guidelines for the management of patients with ST-elevation myocardial infarction – executive summary. A report of the American College of Cardiology/American Heart Association Task Force on Practice Guidelines (Writing Committee to revise the 1999 guidelines for the management of patients with acute myocardial infarction). J Am Coll Cardiol 2004; 44:671–719.

38. Van de Werf F, Ardissino D, Betriu A et al. Management of acute myocardial infarction in patients presenting with ST-segment elevation. The Task Force on the Management of Acute Myocardial Infarction of the European Society of Cardiology. Eur Heart J 2003; 24:28–66.

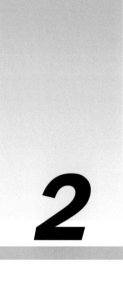

Comparative pharmacology of angiotensin II (AT₁) receptor antagonists

Peter A van Zwieten

2

Introduction

It has long been recognized that the suppression of the renin–angiotensin system (RAS) would be desirable from a therapeutic point of view in conditions such as hypertension and congestive heart failure. Angiotensin II, the major effector peptide of the RAS, has several detrimental actions, such as vasoconstriction and a rise in blood pressure, enhanced release of aldosterone from the adrenal cortex, retention of sodium and water via the kidney, synergistic activity with respect to the catecholamines (norepinephrine, epinephrine) released by sympathetic neurons, and the stimulation of cell proliferation, left ventricular and vascular hypertrophy.[1–3] Several possibilities aimed at suppressing these deleterious activities have been explored.

Angiotensin converting enzyme inhibitors

The inhibitors of angiotensin I converting enzyme (ACE) inhibit the enzymatic conversion of the inactive decapeptide angiotensin I into the active octapeptide angiotensin II (Figure 2.1). The ACE inhibitors, which impair the biosynthesis of angiotensin II, have become successful drugs in the treatment of essential hypertension and congestive heart failure. A possible limitation to their therapeutic use is the fact that they do not completely suppress the formation of angiotensin II. Other enzymes (e.g. chymase in the human heart) also catalyze the formation of angiotensin II, but they are not blocked by ACE inhibitors.[4] Cough is a well-known side effect of ACE inhibitors; it is observed in 10–15% of patients and therefore is a significant drawback to treatment using these drugs.

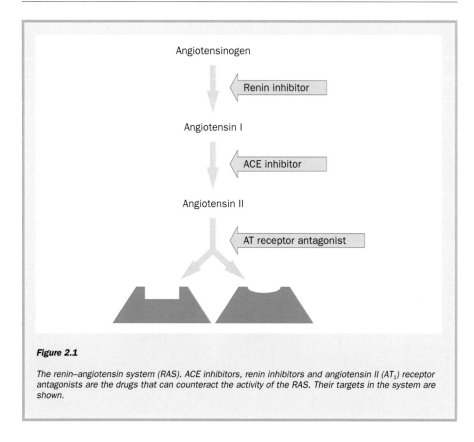

Figure 2.1

The renin–angiotensin system (RAS). ACE inhibitors, renin inhibitors and angiotensin II (AT$_1$) receptor antagonists are the drugs that can counteract the activity of the RAS. Their targets in the system are shown.

Renin inhibitors

A second potential possibility of suppressing the biosynthesis of angiotensin II is offered by inhibition of the enzyme renin, which catalyzes the formation of angiotensin I from the substrate angiotensinogen. Such compounds, called renin inhibitors, will therefore inhibit the biosynthesis of angiotensin II at a site in the RAS which is different from that acted upon by ACE inhibitors. A potential advantage of such compounds is the reduction of plasma renin levels, in contrast to the ACE inhibitors, which cause a rise in plasma renin via a feedback mechanism. Renin inhibitors are indeed available as experimental compounds.[5] However most of the compounds so far developed are rather large, peptide-like molecules with an unfavorable pharmacokinetic profile, which makes them unsuitable for long-term oral therapy.

Aliskiren[6] has been introduced recently as an orally effective renin inhibitor, which, as an antihypertensive agent, can be used once daily. Aliskiren appears to be as effective as the AT$_1$ receptor antagonist irbesartan.

Angiotensin II receptor antagonists

These offer a further possibility to counteract the detrimental effects of angiotensin II. All of these already-mentioned effects of angiotensin in the cardiovascular and nervous systems are known to be mediated by angiotensin receptors of the AT$_1$ subtype. Since the 1970s several peptidergic angiotensin II receptor antagonists have been synthesized and some of them have been made available for research purposes, such as saralasin, sarile, and sarmesin. Saralasin was shown to antagonize the pressor effects of angiotensin II in rats and to lower blood pressure in renin-dependent hypertensive patients and animals.[7] However, the therapeutic potential of these peptide antagonists is greatly hampered by their low bioavailability, short duration of action, and partial agonistic activity.

A major improvement had been obtained by the development of nonpeptidergic angiotensin II receptor antagonists, of which losartan had become the prototype. Losartan was developed by Timmermans and his co-workers[8–10] on the basis of the inhibitory effects of some of the imidazole analogues (S8307 and S8308) against angiotensin II induced vasoconstriction.[11] The basic chemical structure of these compounds led to the development of losartan, which is now appreciated as an effective antihypertensive with a long duration of action, a favorable side-effect profile (no provocation of cough), and satisfactory oral bioavailability. Subsequently, the clinical experience with losartan has been greatly extended, including its potential applicability in the treatment of congestive heart failure.

Several new angiotensin II receptor antagonists have been introduced and clinically developed in the course of the last decade, and many more such agents may be anticipated. A comparison of the newer agents with losartan, limited to those compounds which have been evaluated clinically and then registered, will be the subject of this chapter.

General characteristics of AT$_1$ receptor antagonists

The introduction of losartan as a nonpeptidergic AT$_1$ receptor antagonist has been followed up by an impressive series of compounds with comparable pharmacological and chemical properties.[12] The following AT$_1$ 'blockers' have been developed clinically and registered as antihypertensive drugs in various countries: losartan, irbesartan, valsartan, candesartan, telmisartan, eprosartan, and olmesartan.

The profile of these individual compounds will be briefly characterized below. The common properties of the registered angiotensin receptor antagonists are summarized in general terms below. Some of these aspects merit more detailed discussion, which they receive later in this chapter.

Chemical structures

As shown in Figure 2.2, the majority of the registered angiotensin II receptor antagonists possess a biphenyl component, with the exception of eprosartan. Lasartan, irbesartan, olmesartan, and eprosartan contain an imidazole substituent. In candesartan and telmisartan this imidazole moiety is condensated with a phenyl ring. A tetrazolium component was initially thought to be essential, but it is only found in losartan, candesartan, olmesartan, and irbesartan, not in the other agents.

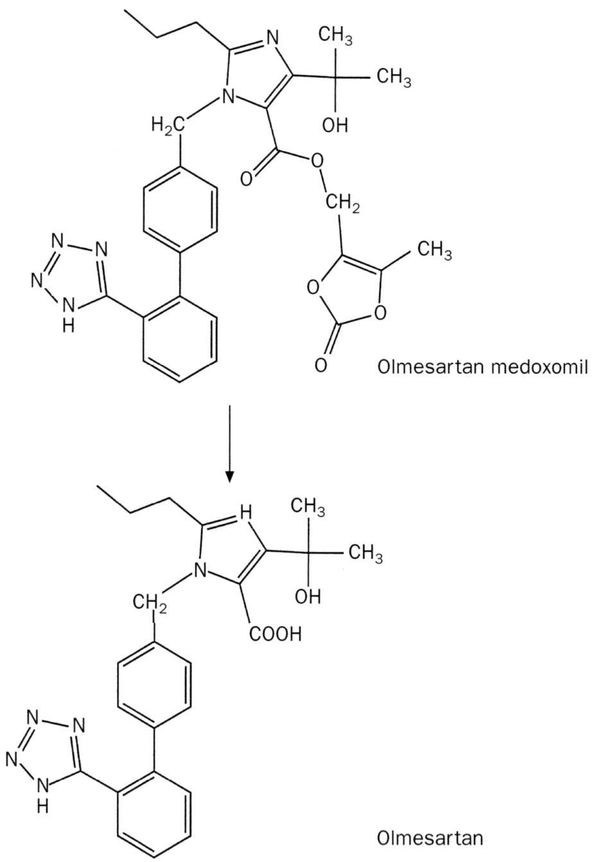

Olmesartan medoxomil

Olmesartan

Figure 2.2

Chemical structures of the AT$_1$ receptor antagonists losartan, candesartan, eprosartan, olmesartan, valsartan, and telmisartan. Losartan, olmesartan, and candesartan are prodrugs, which are converted after oral ingestion into their active metabolites. The other AT$_1$ antagonists are pharmacologically active without modification.

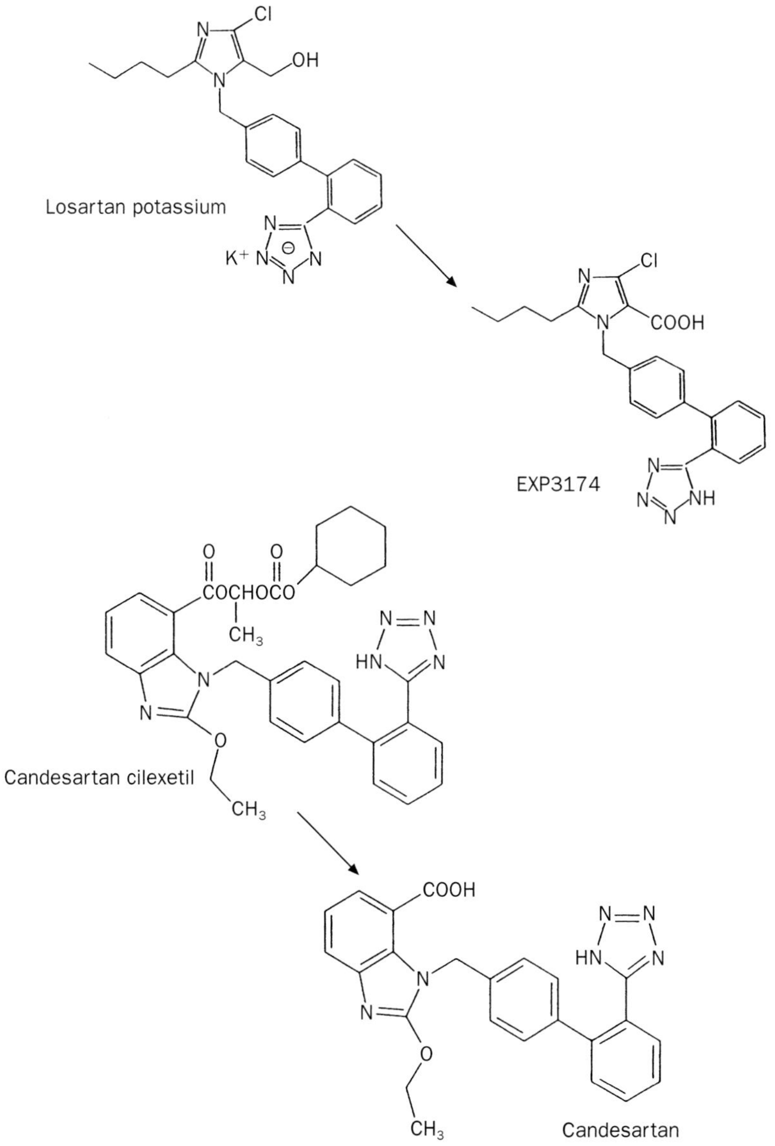
Cl
OH
N
N
Losartan potassium
K+
Cl
COOH
EXP3174
NH
O
O
COCHOCO
CH3
N=N
HN
Candesartan cilexetil
CH3
COOH
CH3
Candesartan

Figure 2.2

Continued

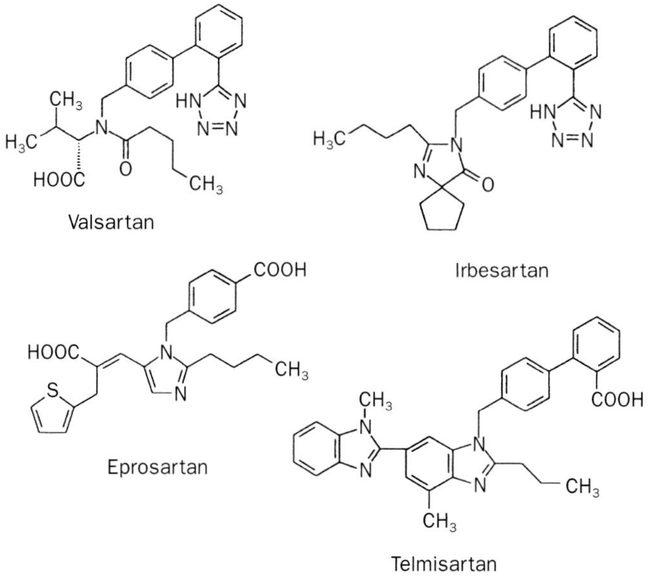

Figure 2.2

Continued

Losartan, a prodrug, is converted in vivo (after oral ingestion) into its more active metabolite EXP3174. Candesartan cilexetil is also a prodrug. In vivo it is converted into its more active metabolite CV11974, the active drug candesartan. Olmesartan medoxomil is also a prodrug. After oral ingestion it is converted into the active compound olmesartan by various esterases.

Receptor profile

Selectivity for the AT_1 receptor with little or no affinity for the AT_2 receptor is characteristic for all of the clinically introduced and registered angiotensin II receptor antagonists.

Type of receptor antagonism

Both competitive and noncompetitive antagonism have been reported for most of the compounds. The issue of competitive vs noncompetitive antagonism, to be discussed later in this chapter, greatly depends on the pharmacological model used and is of little relevance from a clinical point of view.

Kinetic profile

This is discussed in more detail in later sections on individual AT_1 receptor antagonists. In clinical terms, the kinetic properties of the compounds involved are rather similar. All have a long duration of action, thus allowing a satisfactory control of blood pressure over 24 hours after a single oral dose. Most compounds are lipophilic and display a very high degree of plasma protein binding.

Hemodynamic profile

All of the compounds are vasodilators, in particular of the resistance vessels, and hence reduce peripheral vascular resistance.[13] Venous dilatation can be demonstrated to occur, but it is much weaker than the dilator effects upon the arterial system. At the usual dosages, orthostatic hypotension does not occur in antihypertensive treatment. The hemodynamic profile of the AT_1 antagonists is very similar to that of the ACE inhibitors. Heart rate remains unchanged (no reflex tachycardia).

Efficacy in the treatment of hypertension

The efficacy of the various registered compounds as antihypertensives is very similar, although a few reports would seem to indicate that some of the newer agents are somewhat more effective than losartan.[14] This may be a matter of dosage. It is generally felt that the once-daily dose of 50 mg per tablet of losartan is rather low for the adequate treatment of hypertension. In relevant clinical trials, the required daily dose of losartan was in the range of 80 mg.

Side effects

So far, all registered compounds display a very favorable side-effect profile that does not significantly differ from that of placebo treatment. In contrast to the ACE inhibitors, cough is not a common adverse reaction to AT_1 receptor antagonists.[15]

Contraindications

Hypersensitivity, although rare, is a contraindication. Hypotension caused by the angiotensin II receptor antagonists is a drawback in the use of these compounds in patients with hypovolemia (use of diuretics, vomiting, diarrhea) or with symptomatic heart failure. Cautious use is advised in patients with aortic stenosis, renal artery stenosis, or primary hyperaldosteronism. Since data are so far not available, angiotensin II receptor antagonists should be avoided during pregnancy or lactation.

Drug interactions

Used together with diuretics, symptomatic hypotension may be problematic. When combined with potassium-sparing diuretics, clinically significant retention of potassium may occur.

Receptor selectivity

All of the registered angiotensin II receptor antagonists (losartan, irbesartan, candesartan, eprosartan, olmesartan, telmisartan, valsartan) are highly selective for the AT_1 receptor. This selectivity has been established by means of radioligand experiments, usually in the membranes of rat adrenal cortex or hepatocytes. The highly selective affinity for the AT_1 receptor is reflected by IC_{50} values in the range of 1–2 nmol/L. The affinity for the AT_1 receptor is usually 10 000–20 000 times higher than that for the AT_2 receptors, such as adrenoceptors and cholinergic receptors and their various subtypes.

The AT_1 selectivity for the AT_1 receptor implies that during treatment with the drugs the AT_2 receptor is exposed to high concentrations of angiotensin II. The functional role of the receptor still remains unknown, although it is believed to counteract cell proliferation when stimulated with angiotensin II.[16,17] Accordingly, it may be possible that the stimulated AT_2 receptor can inhibit and perhaps even reverse the growth-promoting effects of angiotensin II indirectly, via the blockade of the AT_1 receptor. Furthermore, AT_2 receptor stimulation has been shown to cause vasodilatation in experimental models, thus counteracting the vasoconstriction caused by AT_1 receptor stimulation.[16–18]

Experimental compounds that have affinity for both AT_1 and AT_2 receptors are now available[18,19] but are unlikely to be developed clinically because of their potentially stimulating effect on cell proliferation via AT_2 receptor blockade.

'Surmountable' (competitive) or 'insurmountable' (non-competitive) antagonism

Insurmountable antagonism implies antagonism with a depression of the maximal agonist response. Surmountable antagonism is characterized by a parallel shift of the agonist dose–response curves, without any reduction of the maximal agonist response. These distinct types of antagonism largely correspond (although not in all details) to the processes of competitive and non-competitive antagonism. With respect to the possible clinical relevance of insurmountable antagonism it had been speculated that at high plasma concentrations of angiotensin II (associated with AT_1 receptor blockade) the blockade will not be fully overcome because there is less potential for the increasing plasma angiotensin II levels to overcome the binding of the antagonist to the AT_1 receptor.

There has been a great deal of debate concerning the question whether an AT_1 receptor antagonist is a surmountable or an insurmountable antagonist. This issue requires some critical consideration. First of all it should be realized that the finding of surmountable vs insurmountable antagonism depends greatly upon the pharmacological model used. For instance, losartan is a surmountable antagonist in certain models (e.g. isolated rat aorta; Figure 2.3),[20] but it behaves like an insurmountable antagonist in other models, such as the rabbit isolated renal artery[21] or the vascular bed of the human forearm (Figures 2.4 and 2.5).[22] Similarly, irbesartan may either behave as a surmountable or as an insurmountable antagonist.[23,24] Candesartan has been put forward as a typically insurmountable AT_1 receptor antagonist.[25] This statement is certainly true for a few pharmacological models, but it should be realized that these models are hardly relevant for in-vivo conditions such as the long-term treatment of hypertensive disease.

In conclusion the issue of 'surmountable vs insurmountable' antagonism is of theoretical interest but so far is not relevant for the clinical application of AT_1 receptor antagonists. This issue has been overemphasized for marketing purposes.

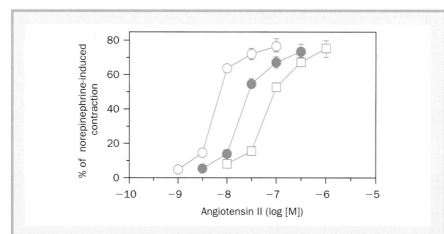

Figure 2.3

Contraction of aortic rings without endothelium (Wistar rats): concentration–effect curves for angiotensin II in the absence (open circles) and presence of 10 nmol/L (solid circles) and 100 nmol/L (open squares) losartan. Points represent means ± SEM (n = 6) of the increase in force expressed as a percentage of the response to norepinephrine (0.3 μmol/L. Note that although there is a parallel rightward shift of the concentration–response curve for angiotensin II, the maximal effect of angiotensin II is nevertheless maintained even in the presence of losartan, thus indicating surmountable antagonism. With permission from Zhang.[20]

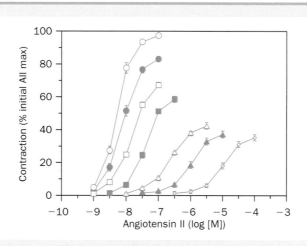

Figure 2.4

Rabbit renal artery: concentration–effect curves for angiotensin II (AII) in the absence (open circles) and presence of losartan at 3 (solid circles), 7 (open squares), 10 (solid squares), 100 (open triangles), 300 (solid triangles), or 1000 (open diamonds) nmol/L. Points represent the mean (n = 5–6, SEM shown by vertical bars) of the increase in force expressed ad a percentage of the initial maximal responses to AII. Note the depression of the maximal effect of AII in the presence of losartan, thus indicating insurmountable antagonism. With permission from Zhang et al.[21]

Profiles of individual AT$_1$ receptor antagonists

Losartan

Losartan was the first AT$_1$ receptor antagonist developed clinically and then applied on a large-scale in antihypertensive treatment. Its safety and efficacy appear to be beyond doubt. Depending on the pharmacological model used, losartan may be seen as a surmountable or as an insurmountable antagonist. A selective AT$_1$ receptor antagonist, losartan is, as mentioned earlier, a prodrug which after oral administration is converted into its metabolite EXP3174. This is a more potent AT$_1$ antagonist than losartan and, in reality, underlies most of the antihypertensive activity of the 'parent' compound.[26] The side-effect profile of losartan is clearly favorable and, on average, not different from that of placebo. The absence of cough is an advantage compared with the ACE inhibitors.[15] Like all other so far clinically introduced angiotensin II receptor antagonists, losartan is therefore well tolerated and accepted by patients. Angioneurotic edema and pancreatitis have been reported in a few exceptional cases.[27] Losartan may also be beneficial in the treatment of congestive heart failure (CHF). In the ELITE-I Study,[28] it was shown to reduce mortality in CHF patients significantly more than the ACE inhibitor captopril. This issue was pursued in the ELITE-II Study, where captopril and losartan did not differ. Losartan may offer some additional metabolic effects that can be favorable. When compared with atenolol in the LIFE-Study,[29] treatment with losartan was associated with significantly fewer cases of new diabetes.

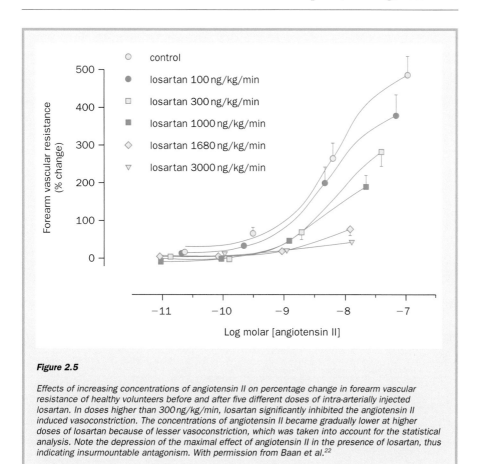

Figure 2.5

Effects of increasing concentrations of angiotensin II on percentage change in forearm vascular resistance of healthy volunteers before and after five different doses of intra-arterially injected losartan. In doses higher than 300 ng/kg/min, losartan significantly inhibited the angiotensin II induced vasoconstriction. The concentrations of angiotensin II became gradually lower at higher doses of losartan because of lesser vasoconstriction, which was taken into account for the statistical analysis. Note the depression of the maximal effect of angiotensin II in the presence of losartan, thus indicating insurmountable antagonism. With permission from Baan et al.[22]

In addition, losartan appears to display significant uricosuric activity in the dosage used for antihypertensive treatment.[30] This effect is limited to losartan and is not a class effect of the AT$_1$ receptor blockers.

Kinetic characteristics

Losartan's bioavailability is approximately 33%. Maximal plasma levels of losartan and its active metabolite are observed after 1 and 3–4 hours, respectively. The presence of food does not influence intestinal absorption. Plasma protein binding is very high (as least 99%). The plasma half-life of the active metabolite is 6–9 hours. The duration of action is sufficiently long to obtain satisfactory control of blood pressure for 24 hours after administration of a single oral dose.

Losartan and its active metabolite are excreted both via the liver and the kidney. Hepatic dysfunction requires adaptation of the dosage schedule. Losartan has been shown to display uricosuric activity,[30] which is not a class effect of the AT_1 antagonists. This may be a potentially beneficial effect when losartan is combined with a thiazide diuretic.

Irbesartan

Irbesartan is an AT_1 selective agent with a long duration of action (at least 24 hours after one oral dose). Depending on the pharmacological model used, irbesartan may behave both as an insurmountable and a surmountable antagonist.[20,21] The side-effect profile does not differ from that of placebo. The occurrence of side effects appears not to be dose dependent. Its antihypertensive efficacy is well established.

Kinetic profile

Irbesartan's bioavailability after oral administration is 60–80%. It is not influenced by food. Maximal plasma levels are achieved 1.5–2.0 hours after oral ingestion. Irbesartan is subject to glucuronidation and oxidation. Irbesartan and its metabolites are eliminated both via the liver and the kidney. Approximately 90% of the administered irbesartan is bound to plasma proteins. Moderate hepatic or renal dysfunction do not require adaptation of the dosage schedule. For reviews on irbesartan, see Gillis and Markham[31] and Man in't Veld.[32]

Candesartan cilexetil

Candesartan cilexetil is a prodrug that, after oral ingestion, is converted into candesartan, the active compound. Candesartan has been put forward as the prototype of an insurmountable AT_1 selective receptor antagonist, but, as such, it is not unique. Its long duration of action (>24 hours) may be partly explained by strong and persistent binding to the AT_1 receptor, but its pharmacokinetic characteristics also contribute to its long-lasting antihypertensive effect. Candesartan is tolerated as well as the other AT_1 receptor antagonists.[33,34] The antihypertensive activity of candesartan is well documented and it has been registered in several countries for this purpose. In the recently published CHARM-Studies, the beneficial effect of candesartan in congestive heart failure has been clearly demonstrated.[35] Accordingly, candesartan has recently been registered in a few countries for the treatment of congestive heart failure.

Kinetic profile

The oral bioavailability of candesartan cilexitil is approximately 40%, and it is not influenced by the presence of food. The maximal plasma concentration is achieved after 3–4 hours. At least 99% is bound to plasma proteins. Candesartan (the active compound) is excreted, predominantly in unmodified form, via both the kidney and the liver. Moderate or serious renal or hepatic dysfunction require adaptation of the dosage schedule.

For reviews of candesartan, see Sever and Ménard[34] and McClellan and Goa.[36]

Eprosartan

Eprosartan is a selective AT$_1$ receptor antagonist. Its binding to AT$_1$ receptors is reversible. Eprosartan may be characterized as a surmountable (competitive) antagonist.[37] Its hemodynamic profile, antihypertensive efficacy, and tolerability are comparable with those of the other AT$_1$ receptor antagonists.

In pithed rats[38] eprosartan inhibits the stimulated release of norepinephrine from presynaptic sites, probably via the blockade of presynaptic angiotensin receptors (AT$_1$ type) on postganglionic sympathetic neurons. The clinical relevance of the inhibition of sympathetic outflow by eprosartan so far remains unclear, although it may be potentially beneficial, in particular in CHF patients, where the sympathetic system is usually activated. It would be potentially attractive to have an AT$_1$ blocker with additional sympatholytic activity. However, for eprosartan such a dual action remains to be demonstrated under clinical conditions.

Kinetic profile

The bioavailability of eprosartan after oral administration is approximately 13% and is therefore lower than that of the other angiotensin receptor antagonists. The presence of food somewhat delays the intestinal absorption, although this appears not be a clinically relevant effect.

Peak plasma concentration is achieved after 1–3 hours. The half-life of plasma elimination is 5–7 hours. Eprosartan is administered once or twice daily. Plasma binding is high (approximately 98%), as observed for the other AT$_1$ receptor blockers.

Excretion of eprosartan, in the unchanged form, predominantly occurs via the bile and feces (approximately 90%), and much less so via the kidney (approximately 10%). Since eprosartan is not metabolized by the cytochrome P450 system, it therefore has a low potential for drug interactions. Severe hepatic or renal dysfunction requires adaptation of the dosage schedule.

For a review of eprosartan, see McClellan and Balfour.[37]

Olmesartan

Olmesartan medoxomil, recently introduced for the treatment of essential hypertension, is a prodrug that is converted after oral ingestion by various esterases into the active metabolite olmesartan.[39,40]

Olmesartan has been shown to produce a moderately rapid decrease of elevated blood pressure. Owing to its long half-life of elimination ($t_{\frac{1}{2}}$ = 10–15 hours) once-daily administration appears to be suitable for blood pressure control for 24 hours. Its efficacy and safety are comparable with those of other AT$_1$ blockers. Large-scale intervention studies such as OLMEBEST are ongoing.

Kinetic profile

The maximal plasma concentration of olmesartan is achieved after 2 hours following oral ingestion. Bioavailability lies within the range of approximately 25%. The presence of food does not significantly influence the bioavailability.[40] Olmesartan is virtually completely bound to plasma proteins. Olmesartan displays a dual mode of elimination and degradation in vivo. Approximately 60% of olmesartan is eliminated via the liver, and the remainder via the kidney. Olmesartan is not metabolized by the cytochrome P450 enzyme system. Accordingly, olmesartan has a low potential for metabolic drug interactions.[39] The bioavailability of olmesartan is increased in the elderly and in patients with impaired renal and/or hepatic functions.

For reviews of olmesartan, see Brunner and Laeis[39] and Unger et al.[40]

Telmisartan

Telmisartan is a lipophilic, selective, insurmountable AT_1 receptor antagonist with a long duration of action. The hemodynamic profile, antihypertensive efficacy, and tolerability are comparable to those of the other AT_1 receptor antagonists. In addition to its hemodynamic activites, which are comparable to those of all other AT_1 blockers, telmisartan displays interesting metabolic properties. In the doses and concentrations used in the treatment of hypertension, telmisartan appears to be an insulin sensitizer, owing to its activation of the peroxisome–proliferator activated receptor subtype γ (PPAR-γ).[41,42] Accordingly, telmisartan's metabolic actions resemble those of the glitazones, such as pioglitazone or rosiglitazone. The value of the combined hemodynamic and metabolic activites of telmisartan is the subject of ongoing epidemiological studies such as ONTARGET and TRANSCEND.

Kinetic profile

The oral bioavailability of telmisartan is 43%. The intestinal absorption is somewhat delayed by the presence of food, but this effect appears not to be clinically relevant. The half-life of elimination is rather long (27–37 hours). Plasma protein binding is high (>99%). Telmisartan is predominantly excreted via the bile and feces, both in the unchanged form and as the inactive glucuronide. Hepatic dysfunction requires adaptation of the dosage schedule.

For a review of telmisartan, see Chrysant et al.[43]

Valsartan

Valsartan is a highly selective AT_1 receptor antagonist that displays competitive antagonism at the level of the AT_1 receptor in isolated issues. Its AT_1 selectivity is higher than that of losartan, although it is unclear whether this is clinically relevant. It can be imagined that the high AT_1 receptor selectivity is associated with a stronger activation of the AT_2 receptor. As discussed previously, AT_2 receptor stimulation is assumed to be a favorable activity, since it brings about vasodilatation and decreased cellular proliferation. In the recently published VALUE-Study, valsartan, used for the treatment of hypertensive patients, was associated with a significantly lower incidence of cases of new diabetes when compared with a β-blocker. Valsartan's hemodynamic profile, antihypertensive efficacy, and tolerability are comparable to those of the other AT_1 receptor antagonists. Valsartan has recently been registered for the treatment of congestive heart failure.

Kinetic profile

After oral ingestion, the absorption of valsartan may be somewhat variable, thus leading to an average bioavailability of 23%. The presence of food appears to reduce oral bioavailability, although this does not influence the antihypertensive activity. Plasma protein binding is high (94–97%). The majority (83%) is excreted in the unchanged form with the feces, and 13% with the urine, whereas a small portion is converted into an active hydroxylated metabolite. Severe hepatic dysfunction (biliary cirrhosis, cholestasis) requires adjustment of the dosage schedule. Renal insufficiency only requires dose adjustment in severe cases who have a creatinine clearance lower than 10 ml/min. The antihypertensive effect is maximal 4–6 hours after oral ingestion, and it is maintained for more than 24 hours.

For a review on valsartan, see Markham et al.[44]

Conclusions and perspectives

The development of orally active, nonpeptidergic AT_1 receptor antagonists is a good example of rational medicinal chemistry and subsequent pharmacological investigation. As far as can be judged at present, the angiotensin receptor antagonists have enriched our therapeutic armamentarium for antihypertensive treatment. They are characterized by a satisfactory antihypertensive activity, acceptable pharmacokinetic profiles, and, so far, excellent tolerability. In particular, the absence of cough is a clinical advantage. Long-term randomized clinical trials are ongoing, and a few such studies (LIFE, VALUE, SCOPE) have demonstrated the antihypertensive effect of the AT_1 blockers, as well as their protective actions on the well-known complications of hypertensive disease. The AT_1 receptor antagonists are of potential interest in the protection against diabetic nephropathy and in the treatment of congestive heart failure, as demonstrated in a limited number of clinical trials. Much more clinical experience will be required to judge the validity of these therapeutic approaches.[45] So far the AT_1 receptor antagonists that have been developed clinically are similar in many respects. Most of them are chemically related (biphenyl derivatives) and selective for the AT_1 receptor. Surmountable or insurmountable antagonism can be demonstrated for some of the agents, depending on the pharmacological model used, but this issue seems clinically irrelevant. Furthermore, it should be realized that the pharmacological models required for such experiments are rather remote from the resistance vessels that are highly relevant in hypertensive disease and also from the target of antihypertensive drug treatment.

In most cases the pharmacokinetic profile of the AT_1 receptor antagonists is satisfactory or even very good, enabling control of blood pressure over 24 hours by means of a single dose. The kinetic differences between the various agents are not impressive and hardly influence the pattern of treatment or the choice of a particular drug. A few newer data, both experimental and clinical, appear to indicate that certain AT_1 blockers may offer metabolic effects that are potentially beneficial.

Many more new AT_1 receptor antagonists are expected to be introduced in forthcoming years, but it seems unlikely that new agents will offer substantial advantages over those drugs which are available at present. It seems more useful to study the clinical benefits of the currently available compounds thoroughly than to design new ones that will probably be very similar or almost identical from a therapeutic point of view.

It can be speculated that the AT_2 receptor may offer a novel target for drug design, but the approach would be directed toward modulation of cell proliferation or metabolic effects rather than toward the lowering of blood pressure per se.

References

1. Goodfriend TL, Elliot ME, Catt KJ. Angiotensin receptors and their antagonists. N Engl J Med 1996; 334:1649–54.
2. Johnston CI. Renin–angiotensin system: a dual tissue and hormonal system for cardiovascular control. J Hypertens 1992; 10:S13–26.
3. Peach MJ, Dostal DE. The angiotensin II receptor and the actions of angiotensin II. J Cardiovasc Pharmacol 1990; 16:25–30S.
4. Urata H, Kinoshita A, Misono FS, Bumpus FH, Husain A. Identification of a highly specific chymase as the major angiotensin II forming enzyme in the human heart. J Biol Chem 1990; 265:22348–57.
5. Kleinert HD. Renin inhibition. Cardiovasc Drugs Ther 1995; 9:645–55.
6. Gradman AH, Schmeider PR, Lins RL et al. Aliskiren, a novel orally effective renin inhibitor, provides dose-dependent antihypertensive efficacy and placebo-like tolerability in hypertensive patients. Circulation 2005; 111:1012–18.
7. Streeten DHP. Outpatient experience with saralasin. Kidney Int 1979; 159(Suppl 9):44–52.
8. Timmermans PB, Wong PC, Chiu AT et al. Angiotensin II receptors and angiotensin II receptor antagonists. Pharmacol Rev 1993; 45:205–51.
9. Johnston CI, Naitoh M, Burrell LM. Rationale and pharmacology of angiotensin II-receptor antagonists: current status and future issues. J Hypertens 1997; 15(Suppl 8):3–6.
10. Unger T, Culman J, Gohlke P. Angiotensin II-receptor blockade and end-organ protection: pharmacological rationale and evidence. J Hypertens 1998; 16(Suppl 7):3–9.
11. Wong PC, Chiu AT, Price WA et al. Non-peptide angiotensin II receptor antagonists. I. Pharmacological characterization of 2-*n*-butyl-4-chloro-1-(2-chlorobenzyl) imidazole-5acetic acid, sodium salt (S-8307). J Pharmacol Exp Ther 1988; 247:1–10.
12. Baan J. Functional role of angiotensin II and AT_1-receptor antagonists in human arteries and veins. PhD Thesis (ISBN 90-9011397-5), University of Amsterdam; 1998:18.

13. Van den Meiracker AH, Admirael PJ, Jansen JA et al. Hemodynamic and biochemical effects of the AT_1-receptor antagonist irbesartan in hypertension. Hypertension 1995; 25:22–9.
14. Burnier M. Angiotensin II type 1 receptor blockers. Circulation 2001; 103:904–12.
15. Lacourière Y, Lefebvre J, Nakhla G et al. Association between cough and angiotensin converting enzyme inhibitors versus angiotensin II antagonists: the design of a prospective, controlled study. J Hypertens 1994; 12(Suppl):49–53.
16. Johnston CI, Risvanis J. Preclinical pharmacology of angiotensin II-receptor antagonists. Am J Hypertens 1997; 10:306–10S.
17. Unger T, Chung O, Csikos T et al. Angiotensin receptors. J Hypertens 1996; 14(Suppl):95–103.
18. Kivlighn S, Zingaro GJ, Gabel RA et al. In vivo pharmacology of an angiotensin AT_1-receptor antagonist with balanced affinity for angiotensin AT_2-receptors. Eur J Pharmacol 1995; 294:439–50.
19. Wong PC, Quan ML, Saye JA et al. Pharmacology of XR 510, a potent orally active non-peptide angiotensin AT1-receptor antagonist with high affinity for the AT_2-receptor subtype. J Cardiovasc Pharmacol 1995; 26:354–62.
20. Zhang J. Pharmacological effects of angiotensin II and non-peptidergic receptor antagonists. PhD Thesis (ISBN 90-9008377-4), University of Amsterdam, 1995; 145.
21. Zhang J, Pfaffendorf M, Zhang JS, van Zwieten PA. A non-competitive type of angiotensin II-receptor antagonism by losartan in renal artery preparations. Eur J Pharmacol 1994; 252:337–40.
22. Baan H, Chang PC, Vermeij P, Pfaffendorf M, van Zwieten PA. Effects of losartan on vasoconstrictor responses to angiotensin II in the human forearm vascular bed of healthy volunteers. Cardiovasc Res 1996; 32:973–9.
23. Cazaubon C, Gougat J, Bousquet F et al. Pharmacological characterization of SR 47436, a new non-peptide AT_1-subtype angiotensin II-receptor antagonist. J Pharmacol Exp Ther 1993; 265:826–34.
24. Délisée C, Schaeffer P, Cazabon C et al. Characterization of cardiac angiotensin AT_1-receptors by [^{3}H]SR-47436. Eur J Pharmacol 1993; 247:139–44.
25. Shibouta Y, Inada Y, Ogima M et al. Pharmacological profile of a highly potent and long-acting angiotensin II-receptor antagonist, 2-ethoxy-1-[2′-(1H-tetrazol-5-yl)biphenyl-4-yl]methyl]-1H-benzimidazole-7-carboxylic acid (CV 11974), and its prodrug, (±)-1-(cyclohexyloxycarbonyloxy)-ethyl-2-ethoxy-1-[[2′-(1H-tetrazol-5-yl)biphenyl-4-yl]methyl]-1H-benzimidazole-7-carboxylate (TCV-116). J Pharmacol Exp Ther 1993; 266:114–20.
26. Dzielak DJ. Comparative pharmacology of the angiotensin II-receptor antagonists. Exp Opin Invest Drugs 1998; 7:741–51.
27. Acker CG, Greenberg A. Angioedema induced by the angiotensin II blocker losartan. N Engl J Med 1995; 333:1572.
28. Pitt B, Segal R, Matinez FA et al. On behalf of the ELITE Study Investigators. Randomised trial of losartan versus captopril in patients over 65 with heart failure (Evaluation of Losartan in the Elderly Study, ELITE). Lancet 1997; 349:747–52.
29. Dahlöf B, Devereux RB, Kjeldsen SE et al. Cardiovascular morbidity and mortality in the Losartan Intervention For Endpoint reduction in hypertension study (LIFE): a randomized trial against atenolol. Lancet 2002; 359:995–1003.
30. Puig JG, Mateos F, Buno A et al. Effect of eprosartan and losartan on uric acid metabolism in patients with essential hypertension. J Hypertens 1999; 17:1033–9.
31. Gillis JC, Markham A. Irbesartan. A review of its pharmacodynamic and pharmacokinetic properties and therapeutic use in the management of hypertension. Drugs 1997; 54:885–902.
32. Man in't Veld AJ. Clinical overview of irbesartan: expanding the therapeutic window in hypertension. J Hypertens 1997; 15(Suppl 7):27–33.
33. Andersson OK, Neldam S. The antihypertensive effect and tolerability of candesartan cilexetil, a new generation angiotensin II antagonist, in comparison with losartan. Blood Press 1998; 7:53–9.
34. Sever P, Ménard J. Angiotensin II antagonism refined: candesartan cilexetil. A novel long-acting selective AT_1-receptor blocker. J Hum Hypertens 1997; 11(Suppl 2):1–95.
35. White HD. Candesartan and heart failure: the allure of CHARM. Lancet 2003; 362:754–755.
36. McClellan KJ, Goa KL. Candesartan cilexetil. A review of its use in essential hypertension. Drugs 1998; 56:847–69.

37. McClellan KJ, Balfour JA. Eprosartan. Drugs 1998; 55:713–18.
38. Nap A, Balt JC, Mathy MJ, van Zwieten PA. AT_1-receptor blockade and sympathetic neurotransmission in cardiovascular disease. Auton Autacoid Pharmacol 2004; 23:285–96.
39. Brunner HR, Laeis P. Clinical efficacy of olmesartan medoxomil. J Hypertens 2003; 21(Suppl 2):S43–6.
40. Unger T, McInnes GT, Neutel JM, Böhm M. The role of olmesartan medoxomil in the management of hypertension. Drugs 2004; 64:2731–9
41. Benson SC, Pershadsingh HA, Ho CI et al. Identification of telmisartan as a unique angiotensin II receptor antagonist with selective PPAR-γ modulating activity. Hypertension 2004; 43:993–1002.
42. Schupp M, Janke J, Clasen R, Unger T, Kintscher U. Angiotensin type I receptor blockers include peroxisome proliferator-activated receptor-γ activity. Circulation 2004; 109:2054–7.
43. Chrysant SG, Chrysant GS, Desai A. Current status of angiotensin receptor blockers for the treatment of cardiovascular diseases: focus on telmisartan. J Hum Hypertens 2005; 19:173–83.
44. Markham A, Goa KL. Valsartan. A review of its pharmacology and therapeutic use in essential hypertension. Drugs 1997; 54:299–331.
45. Weber AM. Angiotensin II receptor blockers and cardiovascular outcomes: what does the future hold? J Renin Eng Ald Syst 2003; 4:62–73.

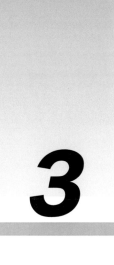

3

Stimulation of AT$_2$ receptors: role in the effect of angiotensin II receptor antagonists

Heiko Funke-Kaiser, Ulrike Muscha Steckelings, and Thomas Unger

Introduction

This chapter will focus on the hypothesis that angiotensin AT$_1$ receptor blockers (ARBs) act not only by blocking the deleterious effects of angiotensin II type 1 receptor (AT1R) activation but also by indirectly activating the angiotensin II type 2 receptor (AT2R). To discuss this mechanism, knowledge about the signal transduction cascade and the cellular and biological effect of the AT2R is crucial.

Signal transduction of the AT2R

The AT2R, which only shares 32% amino acid sequence identity with the AT1R in the rat species, belongs to the family of G protein-coupled receptors (GPCRs) containing seven transmembrane domains.[1,2] Interestingly, the AT2R exhibits some unusual features.

It can display constitutive receptor activation, i.e. intrinsic activity without ligand binding, implicating that the AT2R expression level per se is associated with the level of receptor activation.[2,3] Additionally, the AT2R – compared with the AT1R – exhibits a slower angiotensin II (Ang II) induced internalization, which also does not involve β-arrestin,[4,5] and AT2R ligands seem to prevent AT2R degradation.[6]

Since coregulation of mRNAs and proteins under certain stimulatory conditions does not necessarily imply a causal relationship, it is crucial to identify direct physical interaction

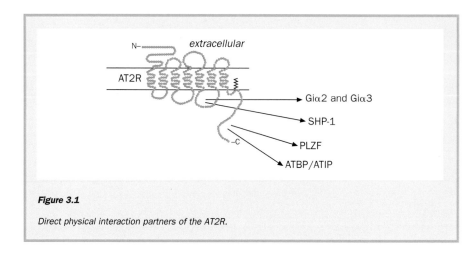

Figure 3.1

Direct physical interaction partners of the AT2R.

partners to clearly analyze regulatory cascades and networks. Direct physical protein interaction partners of the AT2R identified so far include (Figure 3.1):

- In 1996 Zhang et al were able to show that the AT2R couples to both Gαi2 and Gαi3, thereby demonstrating that this receptor is G protein-coupled.[7] Later on, Hansen et al observed that the activation of the Gαi subunit requires the Gβγ subunit.[8] Several studies have observed that Ang II binding to the AT2R was not altered by G protein binding to the receptor, suggesting an atypical role of G proteins in AT2R function.[2]
- Using a yeast two-hybrid screen of a human heart library, Senbonmatsu et al recently identified PLZF (promyelocytic zinc finger protein) as a protein capable of directly interacting with the C-terminal intracellular part of the AT2R.[5] PLZF, which is disrupted in patients with translocation t(11;17)(q23;q21)-associated acute promyelocytic leukemia, is a multiple zinc finger-containing DNA-binding protein normally implicated in transcriptional repression.[9] The authors showed that PLZF can bind to and activate the promoter of the regulatory subunit p85α of PI3K (phosphatidylinositol-3 kinase), causing an increase in p85α PI3K protein level, which was associated with an increase in protein synthesis and with growth promotion of cardiomyocytes.[5] The caveats against such a unimodular function of PLZF are discussed below. Furthermore, p85α PI3K depends for its activation on growth factors such as EGF, FGF, or IGF[4,5] indicating that not AT2R alone is responsible for the observed effects. Interestingly, AT2R interaction with Gi is involved in its interaction with PLZF and in the nuclear translocation of PLZF, linking G proteins and PLZF.[5]
- Recently, it was shown that the AT2R physically associates with SH2 domain-containing phosphatase 1 (SHP-1).[10] However, SHP-1 association with the AT2R and SHP-1 activation required the presence of Gαs alone, rather than the Gαβγ heterotrimer. SHP-1 in turn decreases cellular tyrosine phosphorylation.[2]

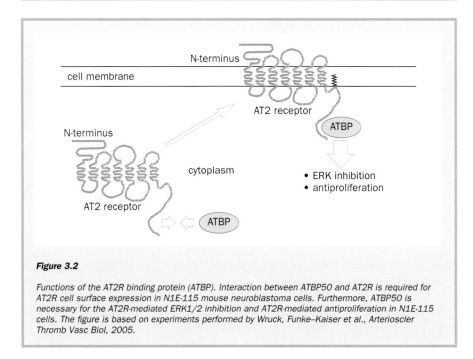

Figure 3.2

Functions of the AT2R binding protein (ATBP). Interaction between ATBP50 and AT2R is required for AT2R cell surface expression in N1E-115 mouse neuroblastoma cells. Furthermore, ATBP50 is necessary for the AT2R-mediated ERK1/2 inhibition and AT2R-mediated antiproliferation in N1E-115 cells. The figure is based on experiments performed by Wruck, Funke–Kaiser et al., Arterioscler Thromb Vasc Biol, 2005.

- Using a yeast two-hybrid screening of a mouse embryo library as a prey, our group was recently able to identify ATBP (AT2R binding protein) as a novel protein that can bind to cytoplasmic C-terminus of the AT2R.[11] Furthermore, the interaction between AT2R and ATBP was verified by coimmunoprecipitation. ATBP is expressed in at least three different isoforms – ATBP50, ATBP60, and ATBP135 – which collectively exhibit a ubiquitous mRNA expression pattern.[11] ATBP50 plays a crucial role in the transport of the AT2R from the Golgi compartment to the cell membrane, and mediates the inhibitory effects on MAP kinases and the antiproliferative effects of the AT2R in N1E-115 neuroblastoma cells[11] (Figure 3.2). On the other hand, AT2R activation increases ATBP50 mRNA levels, indicating a positive feedback loop.[11] Our results on ATBP were confirmed in parallel by two different groups who cloned ATBP-analogous proteins, termed ATIP (AT2 receptor interacting protein),[12] and MTSG (mitochondrial tumor suppressor gene 1),[13] respectively.

Focusing on further downstream localized molecules of AT2R signaling, it has been shown that AT2R stimulation – involving activation of different phosphatases such as SHP-1 and MKP-1 – is able to inhibit MAP kinase (MAPK) activity, which is related to the antiproliferative effects of the AT2R discussed below.[1,14,15] The inhibitory effect of the AT2R on MAPKs depends on the proliferation status of the cellular system used,[16] and was also observed in vivo using transgenic mice.[15] In addition, AT2R activation can also inhibit the JAK-STAT pathway through which certain cytokines and growth factors mediate their effects.[15]

Cellular and biological effects of AT2R activation

Beneficial effects of AT2R activation

It is widely accepted that the effects of an AT2R activation are beneficial with respect to the cardiovascular system since the AT2R counterbalances the growth-promoting, profibrotic, and prohypertrophic effects of the AT1R.[1,17,18]

Using microvascular coronary endothelial cells our group was able to demonstrate for the first time that the AT2R exerts antiproliferative effects that offset the growth-promoting effects mediated by the AT1R.[19] Furthermore, the AT2R exerts antiproliferative effects in vascular smooth muscle cells[20] and pheochromocytoma cells.[21] Growth inhibitory effects of the AT2R were also observed in cardiomyocytes and fibroblasts,[15] which is teleologically consistent with proapoptotic effects evoked by the AT2R e.g. in VSMC, fibroblasts, and PC12W cells.[15,22] In addition, we and others were able to show in neuronal cells that the AT2R not only inhibits proliferation but is also capable of inducing differentiation.[23,24] Consistent with these observations, our group provided experimental evidence that AT2R activation enhances axonal regeneration in different nerve injury models.[25,26] Recently, we were able to demonstrate the neuroprotective effects of the AT2R during cerebral ischemia.[27] In addition, growth-potentiating effects of the AT2R antagonist PD123319, i.e. growth inhibitory effects of AT2R itself, were observed in different in-vivo models, including neointima formation, atherosclerosis, and cardiac and renal fibrosis.[15] Recently, it was shown that transgenic overexpression of the AT2R in the heart preserves cardiac function after myocardial infarction.[28] In a similar approach, AT2R overexpression by lentiviral gene transfer into the left ventricle of spontaneously hypertensive rats (SHRs) decreased left ventricular wall thickness.[29] The renal and pituitary up-regulation of the AT2R by estrogens is also indicative of a vasculoprotective role of this receptor.[30,31]

Detrimental effects of AT2R activation

However, besides the growth inhibitory function of AT2R, there is also experimental in-vitro and in-vivo evidence that AT2R stimulation can promote fibrosis and growth. AT2R activation in AT2R-transfected smooth muscle cells stimulated collagen synthesis,[32] and blockade of the AT2R in Ang II-induced hypertensive rats reduced aortic fibrosis.[33] Furthermore, ventricular hypertrophy induced by pressure overload was not observed in AT2R knockout mice, probably due to the significantly lower expression of p70s6k, a kinase essential to protein synthesis.[34] In addition, some authors observed that PD123319 can prevent vascular hypertrophy.[15] On the other hand, pharmacological or genetic (i.e. overexpression) AT2R stimulation inhibited neointimal growth.[15]

Experiments in AT2R knockout mice

Several papers have been published trying to elucidate AT2R function by performing experiments in AT2R knockout mice. Table 3.1, compiled from Widdop et al[15] and Levy,[35] summarizes these partly conflicting results.

When considering these discrepancies it is important to note that the genetic background conferred by different murine strains might have dramatic phenotypic effects.[36] Consistent with this hypothesis it appears that the beneficial effects of AT2R activation are more pronounced in the FVB/N strain, whereas the C57BL/6 strain seems to be associated with more deleterious effects of AT2R activation.

Furthermore, knockout – and also transgenic – models alter the stoichiometry of biologically relevant protein–protein interactions, thereby influencing the system to be analyzed.[37]

AT2R function in the context of a higher complexity

The discrepancies as regards the functional role of the AT2R discussed above may also be resolved by a model in which not the receptor per se is 'good' or 'evil' but in which the type of adaptor protein recruited to the receptor determines the cellular effects (Figure 3.3). In this context it is important to note that ATBP – also known as ATIP and MTSG, since it was cloned independently by three different groups – mediates antiproliferative effects. Furthermore, it should be mentioned that PLZF can also exert antiproliferative and proapoptotic functions (in addition to the functions described above).[9,46]

Interestingly, a high level of PLZF expression was especially observed in the heart by Northern blotting,[5] which, considering that PLZF might be regulated depending on the genetic background and the (patho)physiological state, could explain the discrepancies in AT2R function observed in this organ. Furthermore, the cellular effects of PLZF are modulated by the presence or absence of growth factors, as discussed above and illustrated in Figure 3.3.

Concerning 'membrane' adaptors of the AT2R, AT1R–AT2R heterodimers have been described which antagonize the AT1R function.[47] In this context it is of interest to note that the AT1R can also form heterodimers with the bradykinin B_2 receptor, which is involved in the pathophysiology of pre-eclampsia,[48] and (catalyzed by factor XIIIA transglutaminase) covalent homodimers implicated in essential hypertension.[49]

Further complexity arises from the fact that AT1R and AT2R are not the only receptors of the renin–angiotensin system (RAS):

1. Ang-(1-7), which differs from Ang II by only one amino acid, can be generated from Ang II by angiotensin-converting enzyme 2 (ACE2) and from Ang I by, for example, neprilysin

Table 3.1
Studies in AT2R knockout mice.

Authors	Strain	Experimental intervention	Cardiac function	Vascular function
Akishita et al[38]	FVB/N	Nonconstricting femoral artery cuff to stimulate vascular inflammation	–	AT2R inhibits SMC proliferation and arterial thickening
Wu et al[39]	FVB/N	Femoral artery cuff	–	AT2R inhibits neointima formation
Akishita et al[40]	FVB/N	Aortic banding	No effect of the AT2R	AT2R inhibits arterial thickening and perivascular fibrosis
Wu et al[41]	FVB/N	Aortic banding	No effect of the AT2R	AT2R inhibits arterial thickening and perivascular fibrosis
Senbonmatsu et al[34]	C57BL/6	Aortic banding	AT2R mediates cardiac hypertrophy	–
Ichihara et al[42]	C57BL/6	Ang II infusion	AT2R mediates left ventricular (LV) hypertrophy and cardiac fibrosis	AT2R stimulates perivascular fibrosis
Ichihara et al[43]	C57BL/6	Myocardial infarction (1 week)	AT2R mediates cardiac fibrosis but protects against cardiac rupture	–
Oishi et al[44]	FVB/N	Myocardial infarction (2 weeks)	AT2R function reduces LV dilation, LV weight, and mortality; no effect on cardiac rupture	–
Xu et al[45]	C57BL/6	Myocardial infarction (24 weeks)	No effect of the AT2R	–

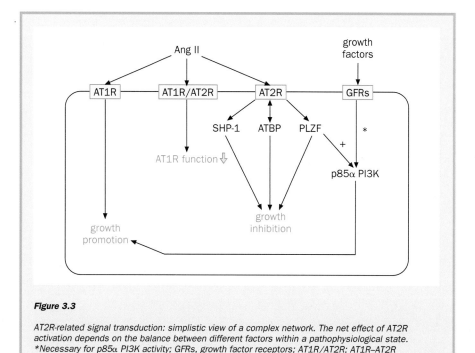

Figure 3.3

AT2R-related signal transduction: simplistic view of a complex network. The net effect of AT2R activation depends on the balance between different factors within a pathophysiological state. *Necessary for p85α PI3K activity; GFRs, growth factor receptors; AT1R/AT2R; AT1R–AT2R heterodimers.

(NEP), and binds to a specific G protein-coupled receptor named Mas.[50–52] Ang-(1-7) attenuates proliferation of vascular smooth muscle cells in vitro and in vivo after vascular injury.[53,54] Furthermore, Ang-(1-7) seems to inhibit hypertrophy of cardiomyocytes and hyperplasia in cardiac fibroblasts.[51] Interestingly, ARBs increase endogenous plasma Ang-(1-7), thereby possibly contributing to the antiproliferative effects of these agents.[54]

2. The hexapeptide Ang IV [= Ang II(3-8)] is a further proteolytic degradation product of Ang II which can bind to the AT4R.[1] This receptor is not specific for Ang IV since LVV-hemorphin-7 is also capable of binding.[1,55] The AT4R exhibits a broad tissue distribution (e.g. brain, kidney, lung, and heart), and does not belong to the serpentine, G protein-linked receptor family.[1,55] The Ang IV/AT4 system is functionally linked to vasodilation of certain vessels,[1] inhibition of renal sodium reabsorption,[1,55] learning and memory processes,[1,55] NF-kappaB activation in VSMCs,[56] and expression of procoagulant molecules such as plasminogen activator inhibitor 1 (PAI-1) in endothelial cells.[2]

The role of the AT2R in AT1R blockade

ARBs are an effective treatment for hypertension, heart failure, and renal end-organ damage.[57] In the following section we will discuss the hypothesis that increased activation of the AT2R in

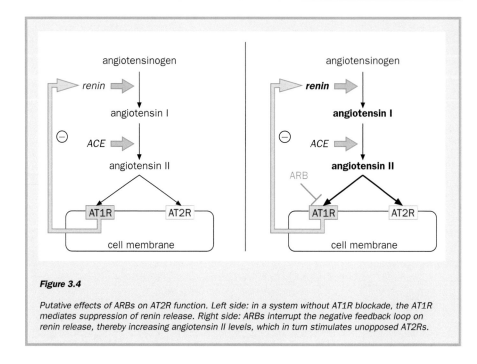

Figure 3.4

Putative effects of ARBs on AT2R function. Left side: in a system without AT1R blockade, the AT1R mediates suppression of renin release. Right side: ARBs interrupt the negative feedback loop on renin release, thereby increasing angiotensin II levels, which in turn stimulates unopposed AT2Rs.

the presence of ARBs contributes to the beneficial effects of these substances on blood pressure and remodeling. Since AT1R blockade interrupts the negative feedback of Ang II on renin release, treatment with ARBs will lead to pronounced increases in plasma, and possibly also tissue Ang II levels.[17] Because this Ang II cannot bind to the blocked AT1Rs, it stimulates unopposed AT2Rs (Figure 3.4).

In this context it is important to shortly address the (co)expression pattern of AT1Rs and AT2Rs in certain tissues which probably – besides the endocrine action of ARBs on the Ang II plasma level – facilitates the functional interaction between AT1R antagonists and the AT2R. AT2Rs are abundantly expressed in fetal tissues but are dramatically down-regulated after birth.[1,14] In adults, expression of AT2Rs under normal conditions is largely restricted to adrenals, kidneys, uterus, ovaries, heart, vessels, and certain parts of the brain.[1,14,58] An up-regulation of AT2Rs can be observed under pathological conditions such as nerve injury,[25,59] stroke,[27] skin injury,[14,60] myocardial infarction,[61] and human heart failure.[62] Interestingly, the up-regulation of AT2Rs after myocardial infarction seems to reflect cell types other than cardiomyocytes.[63] Concerning heart failure, it should be noted that down-regulation of AT2Rs has also been observed.[64] In diabetes, an increase of AT2Rs was reported in the heart[65] in contrast to the kidney.[66] Inconsistent results have been published with respect to AT2R expression in neointima formation.[1,67,68]

Albeit the marked AT2R down-regulation after fetal development, coexpression of AT1R and AT2R in the adult is observed (e.g. in brain, kidney, heart, and vessel wall)[1,58] which probably contributes to the interactions of ARBs and AT2Rs.

Role of the ATR2 in vasodilatory and antihypertensive effects of ARBs

The antihypertensive effect of AT1R antagonists may be partially mediated by the AT2R. AT2R-knockout mice exhibit an increased vasopressor response to angiotensin II.[69,70] Furthermore, one of the two initial knockout models also shows a mild hypertensive phenotype,[70] indicating that the AT2R might contribute to vasodilation. Conversely, the AT1-mediated pressor effect of Ang II infusion is abolished in transgenic mice overexpressing the AT2R in vascular smooth muscle cells.[71] Consistently, it was shown that infusion of antisense oligodeoxynucleotides directed against the AT2R into renal interstitium caused an increase in systemic blood pressure.[72] In addition, coinfusion of the AT2R antagonist PD123319 with Ang II causes a higher increase in blood pressure in rats on high salt diet compared with Ang II infusion alone.[73] Experimental studies using aortic rings of SHRs have shown that the vasodilatory effects of losartan in this model are abolished by AT2R antagonism.[74] Different publications were able to demonstrate a depressor response of the AT2R agonist CGP42112 in conscious rats in the presence of AT1R blockade.[15] As discussed above for cardiac and vascular remodeling, effects of the AT2R are influenced by the murine strain used. The same seems also to be true for direct hemodynamic effects, since the vasodilation in renal, mesenteric, and hindquarter circulation in vivo caused by the AT2R agonist CGP42112 – against a background of AT1R blockade – can be observed in SHR but not Wistar-Kyoto (WKY) rats.[15,75] In contrast, in a very recent study it was shown that AT2R activation contributes to blood pressure-lowering effects of ARBs in normotensive rats but not in SHRs.[76] Nevertheless, with respect to the most relevant species, forearm vascular resistance during Ang II infusion in elderly women taking candesartan – which unmasks a vasodilator response to Ang II in forearm resistance vessels – was elevated by the AT2R antagonist PD123319 compared with placebo.[77] In a similar experimental setting, the blood pressure-lowering effects of valsartan in normotensive rats were more pronounced by coapplication of Ang II or CGP42112 over an 8–9 day period, indicating a direct vasodilator action of AT2R without desensitization.[15] Finally, in a developmental context, it is important to note a very recent study that demonstrated functional AT2Rs mediating vasodilation (but also proliferation) in fetal aortas.[78] With regards to the mechanism of AT2R-mediated vasodilation, several studies have indicated a cascade that involves bradykinin, NO, and cGMP.[79,80]

Studies in AT2R knockout mice

Aortic banding experiments have shown that the inhibitory effect of valsartan on coronary arterial thickening and perivascular fibrosis is weaker in AT2R knockout mice compared with WT mice, indicating that these beneficial valsartan effects are also mediated by AT2R stimulation.[41] The dependence of the beneficial valsartan effect on the presence of AT2Rs was also shown by Wu et al[39] in a model of neointima formation in AT2R knockout mice.

In addition, Xu et al were able to demonstrate that valsartan – in contrast to an ACE inhibitor – increased cardiac function and decreased cardiac interstitial collagen deposition after induction of myocardial infarction (MI) to a greater extent in WT mice compared with AT2R knockout mice, supporting the hypothesis that the cardioprotective effects of ARBs are partially mediated by AT2R activation.[45] Interestingly, as shown in Table 3.1, deletion of the AT2R per se had no effect on basal cardiac function and remodeling after MI in this model,[45] indicating that AT2R function might be linked to ARB therapy (where Ang II levels are increased) rather than cardiac pathophysiology.

ARBs and AT2Rs: further studies

It was already shown in 1997 in a rat heart failure model that the beneficial effects of AT1R antagonism with respect to left ventricular end-diastolic volume and cardiac hypertrophy are triggered by AT2R activation, since AT2R antagonisms with PD123319 reversed these changes (so-called 'PD reversal').[81] Contribution of AT2R activation in effects of ARBs was also described in a pig myocardial infarction model.[82] In addition, a PD reversal has been seen in SHRs examining cardiac fibrosis.[83] Nevertheless, it should be mentioned that a PD123319 reversal was not consistently observed with respect to, for example, blood pressure regulation.[15] On the other hand, it was shown that valsartan induces apoptosis of aortic SMCs and reduces aortic mass in SHRs.[84] These effects were prevented by the AT2R antagonist PD123319, whereas PD123319 given alone had no effect. Furthermore, our group was able to show that losartan plus Ang II significantly increased aortic cGMP content in vivo. Interestingly, this effect was blocked by an AT2R blocker.[80]

AT1R–AT2R interactions and gene regulation

Besides the functional interaction between AT1Rs and AT2Rs described above (i.e. stimulation of unopposed AT2Rs by Ang II) both receptors also interact on the gene regulation level. AT1R activation enhances AT2R mRNA degradation, whereas AT2R activation increases AT2R mRNA transcription.[18,85] On the other hand, AT1R expression is increased on the mRNA and protein level in the aorta from AT2R knockout mice[86] and transfection of VSMC with the AT2R gene results in the decreased expression of AT1R mRNA and protein,[87] indicating a reciprocal cross-talk between these two receptors. Consistent with these observations, Ang II infusion can decrease and also increase AT2R expression depending on the vascular system, probably related to the relative AT1R–AT2R expression.[15] Furthermore, it was shown in endothelial cells that an ARB can increase promoter activity and mRNA of the AT2R.[88] In addition, using a differential display approach, our group was able to show that AT2R activation regulates the mRNA levels of the AT2R itself and the zinc finger homeodomain enhancer-binding protein Zfhep.[89] Interestingly, the sign (i.e. up-regulation vs down-regulation) of this regulation depends on the presence or absence of EGF in this study. In this context it should be mentioned that AT2R activation also up-regulates thrombospondin-1 in endothelial cells.[90]

AT1R-independent effects of ARBs

Recently, our group was able to identify a novel mechanism of ARB action. Certain ARBs, such as irbesartan and telmisartan, but not eprosartan, can induce PPAR-γ activity independent of their AT1R blocking actions, thereby acting similar to glitazones.[91] This observation could explain the insulin-sensitizing effects of ARBs. Furthermore, AT2R activation can induce mRNA, protein, and activity of a PPAR-γ isoform in pheochromocytoma cells,[92] indicating synergistic effects of AT2R activation and PPAR-γ-stimulating ARBs. This synergy is consistent with a very recent observation that stimulation of AT2Rs and also certain ARBs (e.g. telmisartan) can induce adiponectin, which improves insulin sensitivity, in adipocytes.[93]

Conclusion and future perspective

Several lines of evidence strongly support the concept that stimulation of AT2Rs during AT1R blockade contributes to the acute (i.e. decrease in blood pressure) and chronic (e.g. reduction of cardiac hypertrophy and perivascular fibrosis) beneficial effects of ARBs. It is important to note that AT2R expression, which is regulated – absolutely and relatively to the AT1R – depending on the pathological state as discussed above, is a prerequisite for this concept. The variable AT1R–AT2R expression ratios might also explain experimental discrepancies observed in different murine strains.

This view is consistent with a recent publication by You et al.[94] The authors observed that AT2R stimulation (induced by angiotensin II in the presence of candesartan) caused vasodilation in normotensive WKY rats – which seems not to involve cyclic GMP production[95] – but vasoconstriction in hypertensive SHRs. When the mean blood pressure was reduced to 105 mmHg by hydralazine in SHRs, these animals exhibited an AT2R-mediated vasodilation. Furthermore, it was shown that blood pressure reduction in SHRs was associated with an increase in AT2R protein expression in resistance arteries.

Examination of AT2R effects may also be biased by a variety of experimental models with, for example, different drug dosages, treatment length, and 'end point' detection methods (e.g. fibrotic indices). The partly contradictory observations could also indicate that the role of the AT2R per se is neither purely 'good' nor 'evil'. As discussed above, the type of adaptor protein recruited to the AT2R might be crucial (see Figure 3.3). The 'yin yang' nature of the AT2R seems also to operate in atherogenesis, as discussed recently.[96]

The role of the AT2R as a direct therapeutic target might be promoted in the future by the recently described first selective AT2R agonist, 'compound 21', which exhibits a bioavailability of 20–30% and which can lower blood pressure in SHR.[97] Clinically applicable AT2R agonists might also address the problem that the role of the AT2R under ARB therapy is difficult to examine in the human situation. Even the greater benefit of an ARB–ACE inhibitor combination compared with a monotherapy, as apparently shown in the RESOLVD,[98] Val-HeFT,[99] and CHARM[100] studies for congestive heart failure and perhaps in the ONTARGET/TRANSCEND trial,[101] does not allow us to draw conclusions on the therapeutic role of the AT2R, since no data on AT2R function (e.g. mRNA quantification in different organs or effects of simultanous AT2R blockade) were obtained in human clinical studies. As regards the apparent beneficial effects of an ARB–ACE inhibitor combination, it should be mentioned that there is hardly a study in which a high-dose ARB regimen is compared with a high-dose ARB–ACE inhibitor combination.

We would like to conclude with the fascinating observation that lifelong treatment of stroke-prone spontaneously hypertensive rats with an ARB doubles the life span compared with placebo,[102] which putatively also involves AT2Rs, considering the discussion above.

References

1. de Gasparo M, Catt KJ, Inagami T, Wright JW, Unger T. International union of pharmacology. XXIII. The angiotensin II receptors. Pharmacol Rev 2000; 52:415–72.
2. Berk BC. Angiotensin type 2 receptor (AT2R): a challenging twin. Sci STKE 2003; 2003:PE16.
3. Rang HP, Dale MM, Ritter JM, Moore PK. Pharmacology. Edinburgh: Churchill Livingstone, 2003.
4. Landon EJ, Inagami T. Beyond the G protein: the saga of the type 2 angiotensin II receptor. Arterioscler Thromb Vasc Biol 2005; 25:15–16.
5. Senbonmatsu T, Saito T, Landon EJ et al. A novel angiotensin II type 2 receptor signaling pathway: possible role in cardiac hypertrophy. EMBO J 2003; 22:6471–82.
6. Csikos T, Balmforth AJ, Grojec M et al. Angiotensin AT2 receptor degradation is prevented by ligand occupation. Biochem Biophys Res Commun 1998; 243:142–7.
7. Zhang J, Pratt RE. The AT2 receptor selectively associates with Gialpha2 and Gialpha3 in the rat fetus. J Biol Chem 1996; 271:15026–33.
8. Hansen JL, Servant G, Baranski TJ et al. Functional reconstitution of the angiotensin II type 2 receptor and G(i) activation. Circ Res 2000; 87:753–9.
9. Costoya JA, Pandolfi PP. The role of promyelocytic leukemia zinc finger and promyelocytic leukemia in leukemogenesis and development. Curr Opin Hematol 2001; 8:212–17.
10. Feng YH, Sun Y, Douglas JG. Gbeta gamma-independent constitutive association of Galpha s with SHP-1 and angiotensin II receptor AT2 is essential in AT2-mediated ITIM-independent activation of SHP-1. Proc Natl Acad Sci USA 2002; 99:12049–54.
11. Wruck CJ, Funke-Kaiser H, Pufe T et al. Regulation of transport of the angiotensin AT2 receptor by a novel membrane-associated Golgi protein. Arterioscler Thromb Vasc Biol 2005; 25:57–64.
12. Nouet S, Amzallag N, Li JM et al. Trans-inactivation of receptor tyrosine kinases by novel angiotensin II AT2 receptor-interacting protein, ATIP. J Biol Chem 2004; 279:28989–97.
13. Seibold S, Rudroff C, Weber M et al. Identification of a new tumor suppressor gene located at chromosome 8p21.3-22. FASEB J 2003; 17:1180–2.
14. Kaschina E, Unger T. Angiotensin AT1/AT2 receptors: regulation, signalling and function. Blood Press 2003; 12:70–88.

15. Widdop RE, Jones ES, Hannan RE, Gaspari TA. Angiotensin AT2 receptors: cardiovascular hope or hype? Br J Pharmacol 2003; 140:809–24.
16. Stroth U, Blume A, Mielke K, Unger T. Angiotensin AT(2) receptor stimulates ERK1 and ERK2 in quiescent but inhibits ERK in NGF-stimulated PC12W cells. Brain Res Mol Brain Res 2000; 78:175–80.
17. Unger T. The role of the renin–angiotensin system in the development of cardiovascular disease. Am J Cardiol 2002; 89:3A–10A.
18. Volpe M, Musumeci B, De Paolis P, Savoia C, Morganti A. Angiotensin II AT2 receptor subtype: an uprising frontier in cardiovascular disease? J Hypertens 2003; 21:1429–43.
19. Stoll M, Steckelings UM, Paul M et al. The angiotensin AT2-receptor mediates inhibition of cell proliferation in coronary endothelial cells. J Clin Invest 1995; 95:651–7.
20. Nakajima M, Hutchinson HG, Fujinaga M et al. The angiotensin II type 2 (AT2) receptor antagonizes the growth effects of the AT1 receptor: gain-of-function study using gene transfer. Proc Natl Acad Sci USA 1995; 92:10663–7.
21. Steckelings UM, Bottari SP, Stoll M, Wagner J, Unger T. Repression of c-fos and c-jun gene expression is not part of AT2 receptor coupled signal transduction. J Mol Med 1998; 76:202–7.
22. Gallinat S, Busche S, Schutze S, Kronke M, Unger T. AT2 receptor stimulation induces generation of ceramides in PC12W cells. FEBS Lett 1999; 443:75–9.
23. Meffert S, Stoll M, Steckelings UM, Bottari SP, Unger T. The angiotensin II AT2 receptor inhibits proliferation and promotes differentiation in PC12W cells. Mol Cell Endocrinol 1996; 122:59–67.
24. Laflamme L, Gasparo M, Gallo JM, Payet MD, Gallo-Payet N. Angiotensin II induction of neurite outgrowth by AT2 receptors in NG108-15 cells. Effect counteracted by the AT1 receptors. J Biol Chem 1996; 271:22729–35.
25. Lucius R, Gallinat S, Rosenstiel P et al. The angiotensin II type 2 (AT2) receptor promotes axonal regeneration in the optic nerve of adult rats. J Exp Med 1998; 188:661–70.
26. Reinecke K, Lucius R, Reinecke A et al. Angiotensin II accelerates functional recovery in the rat sciatic nerve in vivo: role of the AT2 receptor and the transcription factor NF-kappaB. FASEB J 2003; 17:2094–6.
27. Li J, Culman J, Hortnagl H et al. Angiotensin AT2 receptor protects against cerebral ischemia-induced neuronal injury. FASEB J 2005; 19:617–19.
28. Yang Z, Bove CM, French BA et al. Angiotensin II type 2 receptor overexpression preserves left ventricular function after myocardial infarction. Circulation 2002; 106:106–11.
29. Metcalfe BL, Huentelman MJ, Parilak LD et al. Prevention of cardiac hypertrophy by angiotensin II type-2 receptor gene transfer. Hypertension 2004; 43:1233–8.
30. Armando I, Jezova M, Juorio AV et al. Estrogen upregulates renal angiotensin II AT(2) receptors. Am J Physiol Renal Physiol 2002; 283:F934–43.
31. Suarez C, Diaz-Torga G, Gonzalez-Iglesias A, Cristina C, Becu-Villalobos D. Upregulation of angiotensin II type 2 receptor expression in estrogen-induced pituitary hyperplasia. Am J Physiol Endocrinol Metab 2004; 286:E786–94.
32. Mifune M, Sasamura H, Shimizu-Hirota R, Miyazaki H, Saruta T. Angiotensin II type 2 receptors stimulate collagen synthesis in cultured vascular smooth muscle cells. Hypertension 2000; 36:845–50.
33. Levy BI, Benessiano J, Henrion D et al. Chronic blockade of AT2-subtype receptors prevents the effect of angiotensin II on the rat vascular structure. J Clin Invest 1996; 98:418–25.
34. Senbonmatsu T, Ichihara S, Price E Jr, Gaffney FA, Inagami T. Evidence for angiotensin II type 2 receptor-mediated cardiac myocyte enlargement during in vivo pressure overload. J Clin Invest 2000; 106:R25–9.
35. Levy BI. Can angiotensin II type 2 receptors have deleterious effects in cardiovascular disease? Implications for therapeutic blockade of the renin–angiotensin system. Circulation 2004; 109:8–13.
36. Horrobin DF. Modern biomedical research: an internally self-consistent universe with little contact with medical reality? Nat Rev Drug Discov 2003; 2:151–4.
37. Weinmann AS. Novel ChIP-based strategies to uncover transcription factor target genes in the immune system. Nat Rev Immunol 2004; 4:381–6.
38. Akishita M, Horiuchi M, Yamada H et al. Inflammation influences vascular remodeling through AT2 receptor expression and signaling. Physiol Genomics 2000; 2:13–20.

39. Wu L, Iwai M, Nakagami H et al. Roles of angiotensin II type 2 receptor stimulation associated with selective angiotensin II type 1 receptor blockade with valsartan in the improvement of inflammation-induced vascular injury. Circulation 2001; 104:2716–21.

40. Akishita M, Iwai M, Wu L et al. Inhibitory effect of angiotensin II type 2 receptor on coronary arterial remodeling after aortic banding in mice. Circulation 2000; 102:1684–9.

41. Wu L, Iwai M, Nakagami H et al. Effect of angiotensin II type 1 receptor blockade on cardiac remodeling in angiotensin II type 2 receptor null mice. Arterioscler Thromb Vasc Biol 2002; 22:49–54.

42. Ichihara S, Senbonmatsu T, Price E Jr et al. Angiotensin II type 2 receptor is essential for left ventricular hypertrophy and cardiac fibrosis in chronic angiotensin II-induced hypertension. Circulation 2001; 104:346–51.

43. Ichihara S, Senbonmatsu T, Price E Jr et al. Targeted deletion of angiotensin II type 2 receptor caused cardiac rupture after acute myocardial infarction. Circulation 2002; 106:2244–9.

44. Oishi Y, Ozono R, Yano Y et al. Cardioprotective role of AT2 receptor in postinfarction left ventricular remodeling. Hypertension 2003; 41:814–18.

45. Xu J, Carretero OA, Liu YH et al. Role of AT2 receptors in the cardioprotective effect of AT1 antagonists in mice. Hypertension 2002; 40:244–50.

46. Shaknovich R, Yeyati PL, Ivins S et al. The promyelocytic leukemia zinc finger protein affects myeloid cell growth, differentiation, and apoptosis. Mol Cell Biol 1998; 18:5533–45.

47. AbdAlla S, Lother H, Abdel-tawab AM, Quitterer U. The angiotensin II AT2 receptor is an AT1 receptor antagonist. J Biol Chem 2001; 276:39721–6.

48. AbdAlla S, Lother H, el Massiery A, Quitterer U. Increased AT(1) receptor heterodimers in preeclampsia mediate enhanced angiotensin II responsiveness. Nat Med 2001; 7:1003–9.

49. AbdAlla S, Lother H, Langer A, el Faramawy Y, Quitterer U. Factor XIIIA transglutaminase crosslinks AT1 receptor dimers of monocytes at the onset of atherosclerosis. Cell 2004; 119:343–54.

50. Turner AJ, Hiscox JA, Hooper NM. ACE2: from vasopeptidase to SARS virus receptor. Trends Pharmacol Sci 2004; 25:291–4.

51. Gallagher PE, Tallant EA. Inhibition of human lung cancer cell growth by angiotensin-(1-7). Carcinogenesis 2004; 25:2045–52.

52. Santos RA, Simoes e Silva AC, Maric C et al. Angiotensin-(1-7) is an endogenous ligand for the G protein-coupled receptor Mas. Proc Natl Acad Sci USA 2003; 100:8258–63.

53. Tallant EA, Diz DI, Ferrario CM, State-of-the-Art lecture. Antiproliferative actions of angiotensin-(1-7) in vascular smooth muscle. Hypertension 1999; 34:950–7.

54. Strawn WB, Ferrario CM, Tallant EA. Angiotensin-(1-7) reduces smooth muscle growth after vascular injury. Hypertension 1999; 33:207–11.

55. Chai SY, Fernando R, Peck G et al. The angiotensin IV/AT4 receptor. Cell Mol Life Sci 2004; 61:2728–37.

56. Ruiz-Ortega M, Lorenzo O, Ruperez M et al. Role of the renin–angiotensin system in vascular diseases: expanding the field. Hypertension 2001; 38:1382–7.

57. 2003 European Society of Hypertension–European Society of Cardiology guidelines for the management of arterial hypertension. J Hypertens 2003; 21:1011–53.

58. Lavoie JL, Sigmund CD. Minireview: overview of the renin–angiotensin system – an endocrine and paracrine system. Endocrinology 2003; 144:2179–83.

59. Gallinat S, Yu M, Dorst A, Unger T, Herdegen T. Sciatic nerve transection evokes lasting up-regulation of angiotensin AT2 and AT1 receptor mRNA in adult rat dorsal root ganglia and sciatic nerves. Brain Res Mol Brain Res 1998; 57:111–22.

60. Steckelings UM, Henz BM, Wiehstutz S, Unger T, Artuc M. Differential expression of angiotensin receptors in human cutaneous wound healing. Br J Dermatol 2005; 153:887–93.

61. Nio Y, Matsubara H, Murasawa S, Kanasaki M, Inada M. Regulation of gene transcription of angiotensin II receptor subtypes in myocardial infarction. J Clin Invest 1995; 95:46–54.

62. Wharton J, Morgan K, Rutherford RA et al. Differential distribution of angiotensin AT2 receptors in the normal and failing human heart. J Pharmacol Exp Ther 1998; 284:323–36.

63. Busche S, Gallinat S, Bohle RM et al. Expression of angiotensin AT(1) and AT(2) receptors in adult rat cardiomyocytes after myocardial infarction. A single-cell reverse transcriptase-polymerase chain reaction study. Am J Pathol 2000; 157:605–11.

64. Regitz-Zagrosek V, Friedel N, Heymann A et al. Regulation, chamber localization, and subtype distribution of angiotensin II receptors in human hearts. Circulation 1995; 91:1461–71.
65. Sechi LA, Griffin CA, Schambelan M. The cardiac renin–angiotensin system in STZ-induced diabetes. Diabetes 1994; 43:1180–4.
66. Bonnet F, Candido R, Carey RM et al. Renal expression of angiotensin receptors in long-term diabetes and the effects of angiotensin type 1 receptor blockade. J Hypertens 2002; 20:1615–24.
67. Matsubara H. Pathophysiological role of angiotensin II type 2 receptor in cardiovascular and renal diseases. Circ Res 1998; 83:1182–91.
68. Viswanathan M, Stromberg C, Seltzer A, Saavedra JM. Balloon angioplasty enhances the expression of angiotensin II AT1 receptors in neointima of rat aorta. J Clin Invest 1992; 90:1707–12.
69. Hein L, Barsh GS, Pratt RE, Dzau VJ, Kobilka BK. Behavioural and cardiovascular effects of disrupting the angiotensin II type-2 receptor in mice. Nature 1995; 377:744–7.
70. Ichiki T, Labosky PA, Shiota C et al. Effects on blood pressure and exploratory behaviour of mice lacking angiotensin II type-2 receptor. Nature 1995; 377:748–50.
71. Tsutsumi Y, Matsubara H, Masaki H et al. Angiotensin II type 2 receptor overexpression activates the vascular kinin system and causes vasodilation. J Clin Invest 1999; 104:925–35.
72. Moore AF, Heiderstadt NT, Huang E et al. Selective inhibition of the renal angiotensin type 2 receptor increases blood pressure in conscious rats. Hypertension 2001; 37:1285–91.
73. Munzenmaier DH, Greene AS. Opposing actions of angiotensin II on microvascular growth and arterial blood pressure. Hypertension 1996; 27:760–5.
74. Maeso R, Navarro-Cid J, Munoz-Garcia R et al. Losartan reduces phenylephrine constrictor response in aortic rings from spontaneously hypertensive rats. Role of nitric oxide and angiotensin II type 2 receptors. Hypertension 1996; 28:967–72.
75. Li XC, Widdop RE. AT2 receptor-mediated vasodilatation is unmasked by AT1 receptor blockade in conscious SHR. Br J Pharmacol 2004; 142:821–30.
76. Duke LM, Evans RG, Widdop RE. AT2 receptors contribute to acute blood pressure-lowering and vasodilator effects of AT1 receptor antagonism in conscious normotensive but not hypertensive rats. Am J Physiol Heart Circ Physiol 2005; 288:H2289–97.
77. Phoon S, Howes LG. Forearm vasodilator response to angiotensin II in elderly women receiving candesartan: role of AT(2)-receptors. J Renin Angiotensin Aldosterone Syst 2002; 3:36–9.
78. Perlegas D, Xie H, Sinha S, Somlyo AV, Owens GK. ANG II type 2 receptor regulates smooth muscle growth and force generation in late fetal mouse development. Am J Physiol Heart Circ Physiol 2005; 288:H96–102.
79. Carey RM. Update on the role of the AT2 receptor. Curr Opin Nephrol Hypertens 2005; 14:67–71.
80. Gohlke P, Pees C, Unger T. AT2 receptor stimulation increases aortic cyclic GMP in SHRSP by a kinin-dependent mechanism. Hypertension 1998; 31:349–55.
81. Liu YH, Yang XP, Sharov VG et al. Effects of angiotensin-converting enzyme inhibitors and angiotensin II type 1 receptor antagonists in rats with heart failure. Role of kinins and angiotensin II type 2 receptors. J Clin Invest 1997; 99:1926–35.
82. Jalowy A, Schulz R, Dorge H, Behrends M, Heusch G. Infarct size reduction by AT1-receptor blockade through a signal cascade of AT2-receptor activation, bradykinin and prostaglandins in pigs. J Am Coll Cardiol 1998; 32:1787–96.
83. Varagic J, Susic D, Frohlich ED. Coronary hemodynamic and ventricular responses to angiotensin type 1 receptor inhibition in SHR: interaction with angiotensin type 2 receptors. Hypertension 2001; 37:1399–403.
84. Tea BS, Der Sarkissian S, Touyz RM, Hamet P, deBlois D. Proapoptotic and growth-inhibitory role of angiotensin II type 2 receptor in vascular smooth muscle cells of spontaneously hypertensive rats in vivo. Hypertension 2000; 35:1069–73.
85. Shibata K, Makino I, Shibaguchi H et al. Up-regulation of angiotensin type 2 receptor mRNA by angiotensin II in rat cortical cells. Biochem Biophys Res Commun 1997; 239:633–7.
86. Tanaka M, Tsuchida S, Imai T et al. Vascular response to angiotensin II is exaggerated through an upregulation of AT1 receptor in AT2 knockout mice. Biochem Biophys Res Commun 1999; 258:194–8.

87. Jin XQ, Fukuda N, Su JZ et al. Angiotensin II type 2 receptor gene transfer downregulates angiotensin II type 1a receptor in vascular smooth muscle cells. Hypertension 2002; 39:1021–7.

88. De Paolis P, Porcellini A, Gigante B et al. Modulation of the AT2 subtype receptor gene activation and expression by the AT1 receptor in endothelial cells. J Hypertens 1999; 17:1873–7.

89. Stoll M, Hahn AW, Jonas U et al. Identification of a zinc finger homoeodomain enhancer protein after AT(2) receptor stimulation by differential mRNA display. Arterioscler Thromb Vasc Biol 2002; 22:231–7.

90. Fischer JW, Stoll M, Hahn AW, Unger T. Differential regulation of thrombospondin-1 and fibronectin by angiotensin II receptor subtypes in cultured endothelial cells. Cardiovasc Res 2001; 51:784–91.

91. Schupp M, Janke J, Clasen R, Unger T, Kintscher U. Angiotensin type 1 receptor blockers induce peroxisome proliferator-activated receptor-gamma activity. Circulation 2004; 109:2054–7.

92. Zhao Y, Foryst-Ludwig A, Bruemmer D et al. Angiotensin II induces peroxisome proliferator-actived receptor gamma in PC12W cells via angiotensin type 2 receptor activation. J Neurochem 2005; 94:1395–401.

93. Clasen R, Schupp M, Foryst-Ludwig A et al. PPARgamma-activating angiotensin type-1 receptor blockers induce adiponectin. Hypertension 2005; 46:137–43.

94. You D, Loufrani L, Baron C et al. High blood pressure reduction reverses angiotensin II type 2 receptor-mediated vasoconstriction into vasodilation in spontaneously hypertensive rats. Circulation 2005; 111:1006–11.

95. Pees C, Unger T, Gohlke P. Effect of angiotensin AT2 receptor stimulation on vascular cyclic GMP production in normotensive Wistar Kyoto rats. Int J Biochem Cell Biol 2003; 35:963–72.

96. Kintscher U, Unger T. Does the AT2-receptor mediate anti-atherosclerotic actions? J Hypertens 2005; 23:1469–70.

97. Wan Y, Wallinder C, Plouffe B et al. Design, synthesis, and biological evaluation of the first selective nonpeptide AT2 receptor agonist. J Med Chem 2004; 47:5995–6008.

98. McKelvie RS, Yusuf S, Pericak D et al. Comparison of candesartan, enalapril, and their combination in congestive heart failure: randomized evaluation of strategies for left ventricular dysfunction (RESOLVD) pilot study. The RESOLVD Pilot Study Investigators. Circulation 1999; 100:1056–64.

99. Cohn JN, Tognoni G. A randomized trial of the angiotensin-receptor blocker valsartan in chronic heart failure. N Engl J Med 2001; 345:1667–75.

100. Young JB, Dunlap ME, Pfeffer MA et al. Mortality and morbidity reduction with candesartan in patients with chronic heart failure and left ventricular systolic dysfunction: results of the CHARM low-left ventricular ejection fraction trials. Circulation 2004; 110:2618–26.

101. Yusuf S. From the HOPE to the ONTARGET and the TRANSCEND studies: challenges in improving prognosis. Am J Cardiol 2002; 89:18A–25A; discussion 25A–26A.

102. Linz W, Heitsch H, Scholkens BA, Wiemer G. Long-term angiotensin II type 1 receptor blockade with fonsartan doubles lifespan of hypertensive rats. Hypertension 2000; 35:908–13.

The use of angiotensin II antagonists in combination treatment of hypertension

Bernard Waeber, François Feihl, and Hans R Brunner

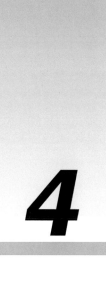

Introduction

During the last decades a lot of effort have been directed to develop new antihypertensive drugs. This has resulted in the availability of a wide choice of blood pressure-lowering agents, the main classes consisting of diuretics, β-blockers, calcium antagonists, angiotensin converting enzyme (ACE) inhibitors and angiotensin II antagonists (AT$_1$-receptor blockers). According to the last guidelines proposed by the European Society of Hypertension and the European Society of Cardiology, these drugs are now considered as valuable options to initiate antihypertensive therapy.[1]

Despite this broad choice of antihypertensive medications, the treatment of hypertension remains a difficult task. This is reflected by the fact that blood pressure is still poorly controlled worldwide, even in industrialized countries.[2] For example, in the United States, only 30% of patients who use antihypertensive medication have their blood pressure normalized ($<140/90$ mmHg).[3] How can these poor results be explained? Are the pharmacologic drugs not effective enough? Are the doctors not motivated to bring their patients' blood pressures down to the target recommended today? Is it a problem related to adverse effects of the drugs, which might discourage the patients to comply with a potentially lifelong therapy? Is adherence to treatment insufficient because of other reasons (poor understanding of the benefits of blood pressure lowering, cost of treatment. . .)? Most likely, all these factors contribute more or less to the failure to control blood pressure in many patients.

Considering the efficacy of antihypertensive treatment, one might expect that any agent administered as monotherapy is able to normalize blood pressure in approximately 40% of patients with mild hypertension.[4] One should keep in mind, however, that the optimal use of most blood pressure-lowering drugs may be limited by the occurrence of dose-related side effects.[5,6] This is particularly true for diuretics, β-blockers, and calcium antagonists, so that dosage increases do not appear today to be the best option when such agents fail to normalize blood pressure. In such a case it has become more acceptable to switch from one drug with a specific mechanism of action to another drug lowering blood pressure in a different way. Another possibility of increasing the effectiveness of an antihypertensive medication is to add a second drug belonging to another class of agents.[5,6] Essential hypertension is a very heterogeneous disease. As expected, therefore, combination therapy, by acting on various sites of the cardiovascular system, improves blood pressure control rates. Generally, full conventional doses of both agents are administered, but low-dose combinations are often effective, allowing us to reduce the incidence of dose-dependent side effects. Fixed-dose combinations are especially attractive in that they are simple to use, and thereby might facilitate compliance with treatment.[7,8]

Ideally, the blood pressure of each patient should be normalized with a well-tolerated drug that has no adverse impact on the quality of life. AT_1-receptor blockers represent an important step in this direction in that they offer a tolerability comparable to placebo.[6] As anticipated, however, blockade of the renin–angiotensin system with these compounds does not normalize blood pressure in every patient. Adding another drug may therefore be needed to achieve complete blood pressure control. In this respect, the most logical combination is that of an AT_1-receptor blocker and a diuretic and a number of fixed-dose preparations containing both types of agents are available.[9,10] AT_1-receptor blockers might also be co-administered with other antihypertensive medications, in particular ACE inhibitors and calcium antagonists. This chapter aims to review the clinical experience accumulated with combination antihypertensive therapy involving AT_1-receptor blockers.

Combination of AT_1-receptor blockers and diuretics

Rationale

The rationale for combining antihypertensive agents relates in part to the concept that the blood pressure-lowering effect may be enhanced when two classes of agents are co-administered.[5] Also, combination therapy serves to countervail counter-regulatory mechanisms that are triggered whenever pharmacologic intervention is initiated and that act to limit the efficacy of the antihypertensive medication. For example, the reduction in total body sodium induced by diuretic therapy triggers the release of renin. Indiscriminate reduction of total body sodium is not always sufficient to control blood pressure and may be useless in some cases. Thus, the compensatory rise in renin secretion induced by sodium depletion is often inappropriately high and may become the predominant factor sustaining high blood pressure.[11] Simultaneous

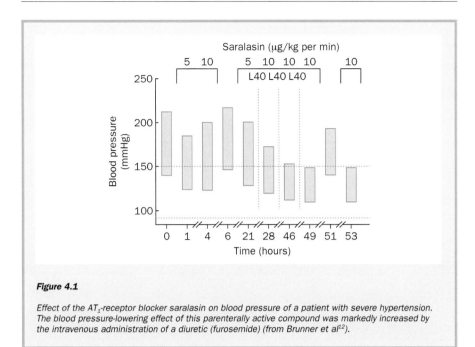

Figure 4.1

Effect of the AT$_1$-receptor blocker saralasin on blood pressure of a patient with severe hypertension. The blood pressure-lowering effect of this parenterally active compound was markedly increased by the intravenous administration of a diuretic (furosemide) (from Brunner et al[12]).

blockade of the renin–angiotensin system makes this compensatory hyperreninemia ineffective and allows maximum benefit from sodium depletion. This close interplay between the renin–angiotensin system and the sodium factor has been first demonstrated in hypertensive patients using the parenterally active AT$_1$-receptor blocker saralasin (Figure 4.1). In this 45-year-old male patient with bilateral renal artery stenosis the efficacy of acute angiotensin II blockade could be improved markedly by concomitant diuretic-induced salt depletion.[12] Saralasin produced a rapid decrease of 15 mmHg in diastolic pressure, but the pressure did not fall below 120 mmHg. However, when 40 mg furosemide (F40) were administered intravenously during angiotensin II blockade, blood pressure decreased to near normal values as cumulative sodium balance was reduced.

Antihypertensive efficacy of AT$_1$-receptor blockade alone or combined with hydrochlorothiazide in randomized, placebo-controlled trials

The interplay between the activity of the renin–angiotensin system and sodium balance was confirmed with orally active AT$_1$-receptor blockers given alone or together with diuretics.[9,10] This can be illustrated by the results of a trial performed using losartan, the first orally active AT$_1$-receptor blocker. Losartan was co-administered with the diuretic hydrochlorothiazide (HCTZ) and compared to losartan alone, hydrochlorothiazide alone, or placebo.[13] A total of 703 patients with mild to moderate hypertension (diastolic blood pressure of 95–105 mmHg) were randomized to a 12-week once-a-day treatment with either 50 mg losartan + 6.25 mg HCTZ, 50 mg losartan and 12.5 mg HCTZ, 50 mg losartan, 12.5 mg HCTZ, or placebo. There

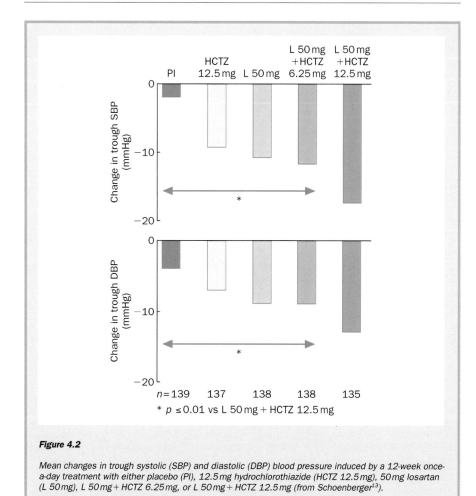

Figure 4.2

Mean changes in trough systolic (SBP) and diastolic (DBP) blood pressure induced by a 12-week once-a-day treatment with either placebo (PI), 12.5 mg hydrochlorothiazide (HCTZ 12.5 mg), 50 mg losartan (L 50 mg), L 50 mg + HCTZ 6.25 mg, or L 50 mg + HCTZ 12.5 mg (from Schoenberger[13]).

was no significant difference in baseline blood pressure between the study groups (around 152/101 mmHg). Figure 4.2 shows the mean changes in trough sitting blood pressure for the five treatment groups. The reduction in both systolic and diastolic blood pressure was significantly more pronounced with 50 mg losartan + 12.5 mg HCTZ than with the other four treatments. The control rate, as defined by a trough diastolic blood pressure <90 mmHg, was 20.9% for placebo, 34.3% for HCTZ alone, 40.6% for losartan alone, and 43.5% and 57.8% for losartan combined with 6.25 and 12.5 mg HCTZ, respectively.

HCTZ has also been shown to increase the blood pressure-lowering effect of the newer AT_1-receptor blockers, including candesartan, irbesartan, valsartan, olmesartan and telmisartan:

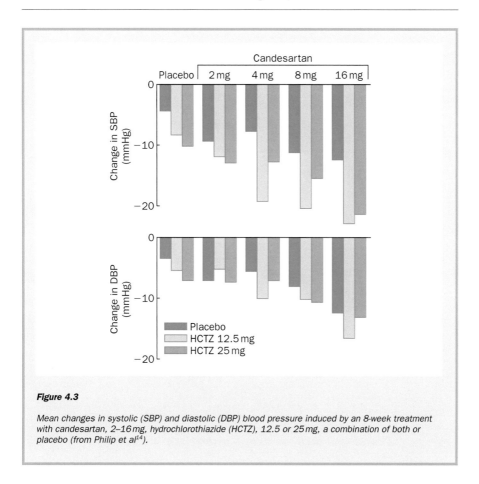

Figure 4.3

Mean changes in systolic (SBP) and diastolic (DBP) blood pressure induced by an 8-week treatment with candesartan, 2–16 mg, hydrochlorothiazide (HCTZ), 12.5 or 25 mg, a combination of both or placebo (from Philip et al[14]).

- In a double-blind trial 1096 patients with mild to moderate hypertension (sitting diastolic blood pressure of 95–110 mmHg) were randomly allocated to once-daily treatment for 8 weeks with either candesartan 2, 4, 8, or 16 mg, HCTZ 12.5 or 25 mg, combination therapy with both agents at these respective doses, or placebo.[14] Figure 4.3 depicts the mean reductions in blood pressure observed during the course of the trial. The greatest blood pressure decrease was observed with 16 mg candesartan combined with 12.5 mg HCTZ. This study suggests that there is no real advantage in increasing the dose of HCTZ beyond 12.5 mg when the diuretic is given on top of an AT$_1$-receptor blocker.
- The blood pressure-lowering effect of irbesartan and HCTZ was evaluated in 683 patients with mild to moderate essential hypertension (seated diastolic pressure between 95 and 110 mmHg). The patients were randomized to 8-week double-blind treatments with various once-daily doses of irbesartan (0, 6.25, 12.5, or 25 mg) combined with 0, 6.25, 12.5, or 25 mg HCTZ.[15] The blood pressure-lowering effect of irbesartan monotherapy was increased in a dose-dependent manner and the co-administration of HCTZ had an

additive effect. At the end of the trial the proportion of total responders (diastolic blood pressure <90 mmHg or decrease in diastolic blood pressure ≥10 mmHg) was 24% in the placebo group, compared with 36–53% in the HCTZ monotherapy groups, 35–58% in the irbesartan monotherapy groups, and 44–80% in the irbesartan/HCTZ combination groups. There was nearly no difference in antihypertensive efficacy between the 12.5 and 25 mg doses of HCTZ when they were given together with the two highest doses of irbesartan.

•   A total of 871 hypertensive patients (sitting diastolic blood pressure of 95–115 mmHg) were randomized to 8-week treatments with a once-daily dose of either placebo, valsartan monotherapy (80 mg or 160 mg), HCTZ monotherapy (12.5 mg or 25 mg), or a combination of valsartan (80 mg or 160 mg) with HCTZ (12.5 mg or 25 mg).[16] All active treatments were significantly more effective in lowering blood pressure than placebo. Table 4.1 depicts the differences between the systolic and diastolic sitting blood pressure responses to all combination treatments and the corresponding responses to individual monotherapies. There was no manifest advantage in terms of antihypertensive efficacy to co-administer 25 mg rather than 12.5 mg HCTZ.

•   A randomized, double-blind, factorial design study was carried out to assess the antihypertensive efficacy of olmesartan monotherapy, HCTZ monotherapy, and the combination of both.[17] A total of 502 hypertensive patients with a diastolic blood pressure ranging from 100 to 115 mmHg received for 8 weeks either once-daily doses of olmesartan (10, 20, or 40 mg), HCTZ (12.5 or 25 mg), a combination of both (10, 20, or 40 mg/12.5 or 25 mg), or placebo. Table 4.2 shows the blood pressure control rate (<90 mmHg for diastolic, <140 mmHg for systolic) observed in the different groups at the end of the trial. The blood pressure-lowering effect of olmesartan was dose-dependent and the co-administration of HCTZ markedly improved systolic and diastolic blood pressure control, the best results being achieved with the 25 mg dose.

Table 4.1
Differences between the blood pressure (BP) responses to all combination treatments and those to individual monotherapies (from Benz et al[16]).

Treatment	Diastolic BP		Systolic BP	
	Difference (mmHg)	p	Difference (mmHg)	p
V160/H25 vs V160	−5.9	<0.001	−10.3	<0.001
V160/H25 vs H25	−6.0	<0.001	−9.7	<0.001
V160/H12.5 vs V160	−4.1	<0.001	−5.6	<0.01
V160/H12.5 vs H12.5	−6.4	<0.001	−10.5	<0.001
V80/H25 vs V80	−6.7	<0.001	−12.3	<0.001
V80/H25 vs H25	−6.0	<0.001	−8.4	<0.001
V80/H12.5 vs V80	−3.2	<0.01	−7.7	<0.001
V80/H12.5 vs H12.5	−4.7	<0.001	−9.2	<0.001

V= valsartan; H = HCTZ.

Table 4.2
Blood pressure control rate obtained with olmesartan monotherapy, HCTZ monotherapy, and the olmesartan/HCTZ combination (from Chrysant et al[17]).

Treatment	Control rate (%)			
	Placebo	Olmesartan (10 mg/day)	Olmesartan (20 mg/day)	Olmesartan (40 mg/day)
Placebo				
DBP	21.4	41.0	53.7	51.1
SBP	33.3	35.9	46.3	60.0
HCTZ 12.5 mg/day				
DBP	35.6	57.1	64.3	73.8
SBP	37.8	60.0	73.8	61.9
HCTZ 25 mg/day				
DBP	37.2	76.3	67.4	79.5
SBP	67.4	78.9	73.9	87.2

DBP = diastolic blood pressure; DBP control = trough seated DBP <90 mmHg; SBP = systolic blood pressure; SBP control = trough SBP <140 mmHg.

- Patients ($n = 818$) with mild to moderate hypertension (supine diastolic blood pressure between 95 and 114 mmHg and supine systolic blood pressure between 114 and 200 mmHg) were included in a multicenter, randomized, double-blind, placebo-controlled trial aimed at evaluating the blood pressure-lowering effect of an 8-week treatment with once-daily telmisartan monotherapy (20, 40, 80, or 160 mg), HCTZ monotherapy (6.25, 12.5, or 25 mg), combinations of these various doses of telmisartan and HCTZ, and placebo.[18] The study groups considered of most interest were the telmisartan 40 mg/HCTZ 12.5 mg and telmisartan 80 mg/HCTZ 12.5 mg combination groups, the corresponding monotherapies, and placebo. Both combinations produced significantly greater blood pressure reductions compared with placebo as well as the respective monotherapies. Observations made using the 6.25 mg and 12.5 mg doses were not reported.

The majority of patients included in the trials described above were recruited in the white population. The observations made in these trials can therefore not be necessarily extrapolated to the black population. African-Americans tend to develop a low renin form of hypertension and are expected to respond better to diuretic therapy than to blockade of the renin–angiotensin system.[19] It is therefore worth mentioning here the results of a 12-week, double-blind, randomized, placebo-controlled trial in which 440 African-American patients with mild to moderate hypertension (sitting diastolic blood pressure ranging from 95 to 109 mmHg) were allocated to a once-daily treatment with either placebo, losartan monotherapy (50–100 mg), or losartan (50–100 mg) + HCTZ (12.5–25 mg).[20] Losartan given alone induced a significantly more pronounced decrease in blood pressure ($-6.4/-6.6$ mmHg) than placebo ($-2.3/-3.9$ mmHg), whereas the losartan/HCTZ combination was significantly more effective in lowering blood pressure ($-16.8/-10.8$ mmHg) than both placebo and losartan monotherapy.

Antihypertensive efficacy of AT_1-receptor blocker/hydrochlorothiazide combinations in hypertensive patients inadequately controlled on AT_1-receptor blocker or HCTZ monotherapy

Using monotherapies it is possible to normalize blood pressure in only a fraction of hypertensive patients. Several trials were aimed at assessing the blood pressure response to the addition of an AT_1-receptor blocker in patients inadequately controlled with HCTZ, or of HCTZ in patients having their blood pressure still high on AT_1-receptor blockade. For instance, candesartan was administered to 234 patients with hypertension unresponsive (sitting diastolic blood pressure >90 mmHg) to a 6-week treatment with HCTZ, 12.5 mg once a day.[21] The patients were randomized to receive for 8 additional weeks either 4 mg candesartan, 8 mg candesartan, or placebo, each in addition to 12.5 mg HCTZ. The combined treatments with candesartan and HCTZ lowered blood pressure significantly more ($-11.0/-7.0$ mmHg with candesartan 4 mg and $-13.4/-7.9$ mmHg with candesartan 8 mg) than HCTZ given together with placebo ($-3.0/-3.0$ mmHg).

The effects of irbesartan combined with HCTZ have also been investigated in 238 patients with HCTZ-resistant hypertension.[22] All these patients exhibited a seated diastolic blood pressure still elevated (93–110 mmHg) after 4 weeks of HCTZ monotherapy (25 mg once a day). The patients were then randomized to receive 75 mg irbesartan or placebo once a day for 12 weeks, with the possibility of increasing the dose of the AT_1-receptor blocker to 150 mg or double the placebo dose at the 6th week if the seated diastolic pressure was >90 mmHg. By week 12, the irbesartan + HCTZ combination had reduced diastolic blood pressure by an additional 7.1 mmHg compared with the placebo + HCTZ combination ($p < 0.01$). Similar reductions were noted in seated systolic blood pressure. A greater percentage of patients achieved blood pressure normalization in the irbesartan + HCTZ combination regimen compared with the control group (67% vs 29%, respectively, $p < 0.01$).

In a double-blind placebo-controlled, randomized trial 328 hypertensive patients who had not reached target blood pressure (defined as a diastolic blood pressure <90 mmHg) after 4 weeks of treatment with candesartan, 16 mg once daily, were allocated to receive for 8 weeks either a candesartan/HCTZ combination (16 mg/12.5 mg once daily), or a candesartan/placebo combination (16 mg/placebo once daily).[23] The additional blood pressure reduction induced by the two treatments was significantly greater in the candesartan/HCTZ combination than in the candesartan/placebo group, with a mean difference in sitting blood pressure of 4.5/2.0 mmHg ($p < 0.05/p < 0.01$).

Another interesting trial was performed in 708 hypertensive patients with diastolic blood pressure inadequately controlled (seated diastolic blood pressure between 95 and 115 mmHg) by

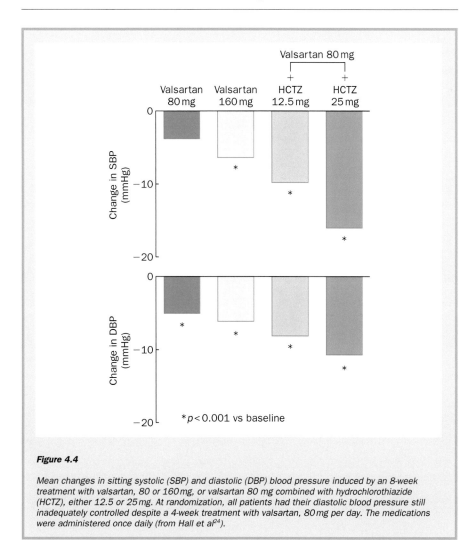

Figure 4.4

Mean changes in sitting systolic (SBP) and diastolic (DBP) blood pressure induced by an 8-week treatment with valsartan, 80 or 160 mg, or valsartan 80 mg combined with hydrochlorothiazide (HCTZ), either 12.5 or 25 mg. At randomization, all patients had their diastolic blood pressure still inadequately controlled despite a 4-week treatment with valsartan, 80 mg per day. The medications were administered once daily (from Hall et al[24]).

a 4-week treatment with valsartan, 80 mg once daily.[24] The patients were randomly allocated to receive for 8 additional weeks either 80 mg valsartan, 160 mg valsartan, 80 mg valsartan + 12.5 mg HCTZ, or 80 mg valsartan + 25 mg HCTZ. All medications were administered once daily. Figure 4.4 illustrates the mean changes from baseline in sitting systolic and diastolic blood pressure. The blood pressure reductions were significantly more pronounced in the valsartan + HCTZ groups as compared with valsartan monotherapies. There was no significant difference, however, between the 80 and the 160 mg doses of valsartan given alone. The best blood pressure results were obtained with the association of the largest dose of both valsartan and HCTZ. Thus, these data indicate that adding a small dose of a thiazide diuretic is more effective in the treatment of hypertension resistant to angiotensin II blockade than doubling the dose of the Ang II antagonist used as monotherapy.

Antihypertensive efficacy of an AT_1-receptor blocker/hydrochlorothiazide combination in comparison with a calcium antagonist monotherapy

Fixed-dose combinations of antihypertensive drugs are increasingly regarded as a valid first-line option in newly diagnosed hypertensive patients.[1] An important issue is therefore the comparative efficacy of AT_1-receptor blocker/HCTZ combinations and monotherapies widely used to initiate treatment. A randomized, double-blind trial was carried out to assess the antihypertensive efficacy of valsartan alone or combined with HCTZ, and that of the dihydropyridine calcium antagonist amlodipine.[25] A total of 1079 patients with moderate hypertension and ≥ 1 other risk factor were randomly allocated to an initial 4-week treatment with once-daily doses of either valsartan 160 mg (Groups 1 and 2) or amlodipine 5 mg (Group 3). At week 4, HCTZ 12.5 mg was added in patients of Group 1 and HCTZ 25 mg in those of Group 2, whereas the dose of amlodipine was increased to 10 mg in patients of Group 3. The second phase of the trial lasted 20 weeks. The diastolic blood pressure responses were of similar magnitude in the three groups. However, the decrease in systolic blood pressure was significantly greater ($p < 0.05$) in patients on valsartan 160 mg/HCTZ 25 mg (-29.7 ± 13.7 mmHg, mean $\pm$ SD) than in patients receiving valsartan 160 mg/HCTZ 12.5 (-27.1 ± 13.7 mmHg) or amlodipine 10 mg (-27.6 ± 13.8 mmHg).

Efficacy of AT_1-receptor/hydrochlorothiazide combinations to reach both systolic and diastolic blood pressure targets

Until recently, priority was given worldwide to the control of diastolic blood pressure. This is because most of the interventional trials that showed a beneficial effect of antihypertensive therapy on cardiovascular morbidity and mortality had taken diastolic blood pressure as both an inclusion criterion and a target.[26] It is therefore not surprising that most trials performed so far using AT_1-receptor blocker/HCTZ combinations have focused on diastolic blood pressure. There is, however, mounting evidence today that increased systolic blood pressure is at least as important as increased diastolic blood pressure as a cardiovascular risk factor.[27] Moreover, it has become clear that the control of systolic blood pressure also provides significant protection against cardiovascular complications.[28] According to the current official guidelines, blood pressure should be decreased to at least 140/90 mmHg in all hypertensive patients, and even lower in hypertensive patients with diabetes or renal disease.[1,29–32] In fact, it is more difficult to normalize systolic than diastolic blood pressure.[33,34]

There is unfortunately very little information available on the fraction of hypertensive patients who actually achieve a blood pressure of less than 140/90 mmHg when treated with an AT_1-receptor blocker/HCTZ combination. Some pieces of information come from the observations made in the LIFE and the VALUE trials.[35,36] The LIFE trial included 9193 patients with essential hypertension (sitting blood pressure 160–200/95–115 mmHg) and electrocardiographically determined left ventricular hypertrophy.[35] These patients were assigned to a treatment for at least 4 years consisting of either an AT$_1$-receptor blocker (losartan)- or a β-blocker (atenolol)-based regimen, with a target blood pressure of less or equal to 140/90 mmHg. In the losartan group (*n* = 4605) the treatment was initiated with once-daily losartan 50 mg, with the possibility of adding (when required) HCTZ 12.5 mg, and then increasing the dose of losartan to once-daily 100 mg combined with HCTZ 12.5–25 mg. The target blood pressure was reached at the end of the follow-up in 49% of the patients in the AT$_1$-receptor blocker group. Notably, out of the patients who were still on losartan at the end of the trial (*n* = 3562), 81.1% were ≥2 drugs. The VALUE trial was a prospective, double-blind, randomized, active-controlled trial aimed at comparing the effects of an AT$_1$-receptor blocker (valsartan)- and a calcium antagonist (amlodipine)-based treatment on the outcome of 15 245 hypertensive patients aged 50 years or older with high cardiovascular risk.[36] The mean follow-up was 4.2 years. A target blood pressure was set at less than 140/90 mmHg. In the AT$_1$-receptor blocker group (*n* = 7649) a once-daily treatment consisting of valsartan 80 mg was initiated, followed if necessary by valsartan 160 mg, valsartan 160 mg combined with HCTZ 12.5 or 25 mg, and finally complemented by other antihypertensive drugs. The target blood pressure was achieved in 56% of this valsartan group. At the end of the trial 3943 patients were still on valsartan, 47.6% of them being on ≥2 drugs. These observations obtained in long-term interventional trials point to the necessity of combining antihypertensive drugs, in particular diuretics, in a large fraction of patients in order to lower blood pressure to the targets proposed nowadays.

In everyday clinical practice a higher rate of systolic and diastolic blood pressure normalization might be obtained by co-administering an AT$_1$-receptor blocker and HCTZ. This is suggested by the observations made in a 1-year open-label study in which it was attempted to bring blood pressure below 140/90 mmHg using a once-daily administration of irbesartan (75–300 mg) combined with HCTZ (12.5–25 mg).[37] The target blood pressure was reached in 65%, 75%, and 70% of patients at months 2, 6, and 12, respectively.

Tolerability

The tolerability of AT$_1$-receptor blockers is very good, practically similar to that of placebo.[6] This is a well-established and very much appreciated class effect. Another classical advantage of these blockers of the renin–angiotensin system is the lack of dose-dependent increase in the incidence of side effects. This allows us to choose the dose of any of these agents large enough to provide a sustained blockade of the renin–angiotensin system without having to worry about troublesome consequences in terms of tolerability. This may be of particular importance when an AT$_1$-receptor blocker is combined with a diuretic, since, in a salt-depleted condition, circulating angiotensin II levels are expected to be high, so that doses of AT$_1$-receptor blockers able to optimally block angiotensin II receptors might be required.

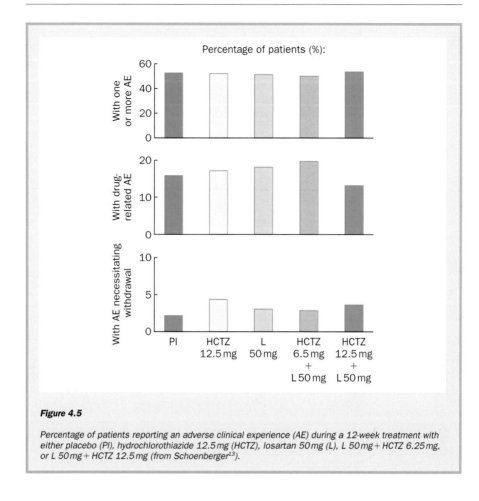

Figure 4.5

Percentage of patients reporting an adverse clinical experience (AE) during a 12-week treatment with either placebo (PI), hydrochlorothiazide 12.5 mg (HCTZ), losartan 50 mg (L), L 50 mg + HCTZ 6.25 mg, or L 50 mg + HCTZ 12.5 mg (from Schoenberger[13]).

Actually, the experience accumulated so far clearly shows that adding a small dose of a thiazide diuretic to an AT_1-receptor blocker has no adverse impact on the tolerability point of view. This is illustrated in Figure 4.5, which depicts the adverse clinical experiences reported in patients having been treated daily for 12 weeks with either placebo, 12.5 mg HCTZ, 50 mg losartan, 50 mg losartan + 6.25 mg HCTZ, or 50 mg losartan + 12.5 mg HCTZ.[13] No difference was observed between the treatment groups regarding the percentage of patients who reported adverse effects, or had to interrupt therapy because of the occurrence of an adverse event.

Metabolic effects

AT_1-receptor blockers have no deleterious effects on glucose homeostasis and lipid metabolism in hypertensive patients, whether they are administered alone or in combination with a diuretic. It is noteworthy that the dosage of thiazides added to an AT_1-receptor blocker can be kept in the lower range, which also accounts for the neutral metabolic effects of the therapy. In fact, AT$_1$-receptor blockade has been shown to improve insulin sensitivity and delay or prevent the occurrence of new-onset diabetes.[38–40] Improved delivery of insulin and glucose to the peripheral skeletal muscle as well as direct effects on cellular glucose transport and insulin signaling pathways might contribute to this beneficial property of AT$_1$-receptor blockers. Moreover, some AT$_1$-receptor blockers, in particular telmisartan and irbesartan, enhance PPAR-γ activity, which is expected to have a positive impact on the prevention of type 2 diabetes development.[41] The favorable effects of AT$_1$-receptor blockers on insulin sensitivity appear to persist during co-administration of HCTZ; a diuretic known to exert an adverse influence on glucose tolerance and incident type 2 diabetes. This is strongly suggested by the observations made in long-term randomized clinical trials comparing an AT$_1$-receptor blocker-based treatment with drug regimens involving no blocker of the renin–angiotensin system. For instance, new-onset diabetes was 25% less frequent in the losartan-based treatment of the LIFE trial, even if most patients received HCTZ on top of the AT$_1$-receptor blocker.[35] In the VALUE trial, the risk of incident diabetes was reduced by 19% by the valsartan- compared with the amlodipine-based treatment.[36]

Thiazides are known to induce a dose-dependent decrease in serum potassium and increase in serum uric acid. Again, because of the low doses of thiazides most often used in combination with AT$_1$-receptor blockers, there are generally no consistent changes in these parameters. The diuretic-induced salt depletion normally leads to a secondary hyperaldosteronism, which in turn enhances urinary potassium excretion. This aldosterone response is blunted during AT$_1$-receptor blockade since all currently available angiotensin II antagonists specifically bind to the AT$_1$-receptor, i.e. the receptor subtype involved in the angiotensin II-mediated release of aldosterone. As an example, the effects of losartan administered on a background of HCTZ on serum potassium is illustrated in Table 4.3. In this trial 304 patients with a diastolic blood pressure between 93 and 120 mmHg received HCTZ, 25 mg daily, for 4 weeks. On top of this treatment they were then randomly allocated to either 25, 50, or 100 mg losartan once a day, or placebo.[42] In this study HCTZ administered alone induced a clear-cut decrease in serum potassium concentrations. Co-treatment with losartan prevented these changes to a large extent.

Table 4.3
Serum potassium (mmol/L, mean ± SD) before the study, after HCTZ, and at week 12 after additon of either placebo or losartan (from Soffer et al[42]).

Treatment	Baseline	After HCTZ	Week 12 (HCTZ and placebo or losartan
Placebo	4.26 ± 0.3	3.92 ± 0.4	3.88 ± 0.4
Losartan 25	4.30 ± 0.4	4.03 ± 0.4	4.10 ± 0.4*
Losartan 50	4.35 ± 0.3	4.00 ± 0.4	4.05 ± 0.4*
Losartan 100	4.26 ± 0.4	4.00 ± 0.4	4.10 ± 0.4*

*$p < 0.05$ vs HCTZ.

Table 4.4
Serum uric acid concentration (μmol/L, mean ± SD) before the study, after HCTZ, and at week 12 after addition of either placebo or losartan (from Soffer et al[42]).

Treatment	Baseline	After HCTZ	Week 12
Placebo	395 ± 89	463 ± 107	472 ± 107
Losartan 25	393 ± 77	462 ± 95	447 ± 95**
Losartan 50	385 ± 95	453 ± 113	437 ± 101**
Losartan 100	378 ± 95	435 ± 101	410 ± 101**

**p < 0.001 vs HCTZ.

During recent years increasing attention has been paid to the effect of diuretics on uricemia. This is because there are indications that elevated serum uric acid may be an independent risk factor for cardiovascular diseases.[43] An interesting feature of losartan, which is unique for AT_1-receptor blockers, is to exert a uricosuric action resulting in a dose-dependent decrease in uric acid concentration.[44] The ability of losartan to increase uric acid excretion is a property of the mother compound and is not observed with the active metabolite E-3174. Losartan reduces serum uric acid by inhibiting an anion-proton exchanger in the proximal tubules of the renal glomeruli, with an ensuing enhanced urate elimination. Addition of losartan to HCTZ allows prevention of the diuretic-induced hyperuricemia. This is shown in Table 4.4, which is also taken from the study described above and involving hypertensive patients having received different doses of losartan in addition to HCTZ.[42] It is relevant that even AT_1-receptor blockers devoid of uricosuric activity tend to lessen the increase in serum uric acid levels due to HCTZ.[15,16]

Combination of AT_1-receptor blockers and ACE inhibitors

Rationale

Theoretically, the combination of an AT_1-receptor blocker with an ACE inhibitor may be of clinical benefit in the treatment of hypertension. On the one hand, some angiotensin II can still be formed during effective ACE inhibition through alternative enzymes such as chymase, cathepsin G, and trypsin.[45] Co-administering an AT_1-receptor blocker appears therefore appealing since such a compound is expected, by acting directly at the AT_1-receptor, to provide complete angiotensin II blockade. On the other hand, ACE is involved not only in angiotensin I processing but also in bradykinin generation.[46] ACE inhibition can therefore lead to some accumulation of bradykinin, a potent vasodilating peptide known to act by releasing NO and prostacyclin from the endothelium. This ACE inhibition-induced decreased breakdown of bradykinin might have positive effects on the vasculature beyond that related to the enhanced vasorelaxation. For example, NO has an inhibitory effect on mitogenesis and proliferation of vascular smooth muscle cells and both NO and prostacyclin can decrease platelet aggregation. Thus, at least theoretically, simultaneous treatment with an ACE inhibitor and an AT_1-receptor blocker might provide maximal blockade of the renin–angiotensin system and optimal cardiovascular protection.

Antihypertensive efficacy and tolerability

AT$_1$-receptor blockers and ACE inhibitors are equally effective in lowering blood pressure in hypertensive patients.[6] When given together, possibly because of achievement of a maximal blockade of the renin–angiotensin system or the presence of an underlying bradykinin-induced vasodilation, the antihypertensive effect is increased. For example, in a randomized, double-blind, parallel group trial, 177 patients with mild to moderate hypertension (diastolic blood pressure ranging from 95 to 115 mmHg) were allocated to a 6-week once-daily treatment with either losartan 50 mg, enalapril 10 mg, or the co-administration of both losartan 50 mg and enalapril 10 mg.[47] The combination therapy induced a supplementary, significant fall in diastolic blood pressure [difference vs enalapril alone = 4.0 mmHg ($p<0.01$) and difference vs losartan alone = 3.2 mmHg ($p<0.05$)]. The corresponding differences for systolic blood pressure were also in favor of the combination (4.1 and 2.5 mmHg, respectively), but did not achieve a significant level compared with the monotherapies.

In another trial 327 patients with mild to moderate hypertension (diastolic blood pressure >95 mmHg and <115 mmHg) received 80 mg once-daily valsartan for 4 weeks.[48] At the end of this initial phase of monotherapy, 153 patients (46%) had their diastolic blood pressure ≤90 mmHg. The remaining patients were randomized to receive once daily for four additional weeks either the ACE inhibitor benazepril 10 mg or HCTZ 12.5 mg on top of valsartan 80 mg. In those patients unresponsive to AT$_1$-receptor blocker monotherapy, the two combinations induced an additional significant blood pressure reduction, which was of similar magnitude for diastolic blood pressure (-4.5 mmHg during valsartan–HCTZ treatment and -3.3 mmHg during valsartan–benazepril treatment). The difference was of greater magnitude for systolic blood pressure during valsartan–HCTZ (-6.8 mmHg) than during valsartan-benazepril treatment, but did, however, not achieve a significant level.

Combination therapy with an AT$_1$-receptor and an ACE inhibitor appears particularly attractive to delay the progression of chronic renal disease.[49,50] At comparable blood pressure, the two blockers of the renin–angiotensin system given together seem more effective in reducing proteinuria than individual monotherapies. This is of critical importance, as proteinuria is a major predictor of decline in renal function in patients with diabetic and non-diabetic renal disease. Angiotensin II contributes to the pathophysiology of chronic nephropathy via both hemodynamic and non-hemodynamic mechanisms. Co-administering an AT$_1$-receptor blocker and an ACE inhibitor may allow us to achieve optimal blockade of the renin–angiotensin system in the kidneys and, thereby, maximal renoprotection.

The AT$_1$-receptor blocker–ACE inhibitor association is well tolerated, but one might expect an increased incidence of the adverse effects encountered during ACE inhibition, mainly coughing.

Combination of AT₁-receptor blockers and calcium antagonists

Rationale

A logical association is that of an AT_1-receptor blocker and a calcium antagonist, especially one belonging to the class of dihydropyridines. The marked vasodilation induced by the latter agents may trigger a reflex increase in sympathetic nerve activity and stimulate renin secretion, mainly during the initial phase of treatment. The enhanced adrenergic state accounts for the transient heart rate acceleration and/or the palpitations occurring frequently within the few hours after drug intake. The dihydropyridine-induced vasodilation is manifested also by side effects such as headaches, flushing, and leg edema. All these side effects have a clear-cut, dose-dependent character and can be largely attenuated using low doses of long-acting compounds.[51] The reflex activation of pressor systems mediated by calcium antagonists as well as the side effects of these agents can be prevented to a large extent by simultaneous blockade of the renin–angiotensin system. Notably, low doses of calcium antagonists generally suffice to lower blood pressure synergistically with blockers of the renin–angiotensin system, which is also expected to have a positive impact on tolerability.

Antihypertensive efficacy and tolerability

Calcium antagonists and AT_1-receptor blockers are frequently co-administered in everyday practice to treat hypertension, but only a few trials have been reported so far to describe the antihypertensive efficacy and the tolerability of such a drug combination.

In one trial 216 patients with moderate to severe hypertension entered a 12-week, open-label treatment period with the aim of bringing diastolic blood pressure below 95 mmHg.[52] The treatment was started with once-daily candesartan 8 mg, increased to 16 mg if needed, and then combined when required with amlodipine 5 mg, followed by HCTZ 25 mg. At the end of this treatment adjustment period, 19.1% of patients were on candesartan 8 mg, 15.4% on candesartan 16 mg, 29.0% on candesartan 16 mg + amlodipine 5 mg and 17.9% on candesartan 16 mg + amlodipine 5 mg and HCTZ 25 mg. Patients ($n = 67$) whose diastolic blood pressure was controlled to <95 mmHg at completion of this phase were randomly allocated to either the continuation of the previous candesartan-based regimen, or the same treatment as before, with, however, candesartan being replaced by a matching placebo. In the patients who had their candesartan withdrawn, blood pressure rose by an average of 13/6 mmHg ($p < 0.0001$) compared with those patients who were still on candesartan. These observations indicate that AT_1-receptor blockade with candesartan used alone or, in most patients, in combination with amlodipine, or amlodipine + HCTZ, represents an effective way to treat moderate to severe hypertension.

Another trial was designed to compare the antihypertensive efficacy of long-acting dihydropyridine calcium channel blockers with AT_1-receptor blockers. A total of 302 hypertensive patients were randomized to a 6-week treatment with either a low-dose calcium antagonist (felodipine 5 mg, amlodipine 5 mg, or lacidipine 2 mg) or a low-dose AT_1-receptor blocker (irbesartan 150 mg, candesartan 8 mg, losartan 50 mg, telmisartan 40 mg, or valsartan 40 mg).[53] The low-dose monotherapy normalized blood pressure ($<140/90$ mmHg) in 53.8% and 55.3% of patients on the calcium antagonist- and AT_1-receptor blocker therapy, respectively. The remaining patients were then randomly assigned to an additional 6-week treatment with either double the doses of the initial monotherapies or a combination of low doses of the initial therapy $+$ a low dose of a drug from the other class. The high-dose calcium antagonist and AT_1-receptor blocker monotherapies normalized blood pressure in 42.8% and 40.5% of cases, respectively. The low-dose combination did significantly better ($p < 0.05$), with a blood pressure control rate of 61.6%. Overall, the blocker of the renin–angiotensin system was better tolerated than the calcium antagonist. Interestingly, drug withdrawal or treatment modification was significantly ($p < 0.05$) more often required among patients on the high-dose of calcium antagonists (11.4%) than among those on the high dose of AT_1-receptor blockers (4.8%) or the low-dose combination (6.7%).

Fixed vs liberal antihypertensive combination therapy

There is no doubt that combination antihypertensive therapy represents an effective way of improving the chances of achieving blood pressure control in the community. Co-administering an AT_1-receptor blocker with a diuretic can be regarded as the prototype of a rational, effective, and well-tolerated combination for the management of hypertension. In some patients, mainly in those with refractory hypertension or impaired renal function, it may be necessary to use a loop rather than a thiazide diuretic. In some cases it might even be necessary to titrate the dose of the diuretic, especially if a loop diuretic is used, so that liberal prescription of the combined agents is indispensable. The risk of using the diuretic component at a high dosage is then to favor the occurrence of dose-dependent metabolic side effects.

Given the current impossibility of achieving strict blood pressure control in most hypertensive patients with any monotherapy, starting therapy with a fixed-dose combination appears more and more appealing. This is particularly true for combinations containing an AT_1-receptor blocker and a thiazide diuretic. Such preparations generally involve a low-dose of HCTZ (12.5–25 mg), and a usual dose of the AT_1-receptor blocker, but can still be considered as low-dose combinations as the placebo-like tolerability of AT_1-receptor blockers is maintained regardless of their dosage.[6] Optimal fixed-dose combinations should meet certain criteria:

- the components should decrease blood pressure by mechanisms that are different and complementary
- the blood pressure-decreasing effect of the drug combination should be consistently greater than that of the components given alone
- the incidence of adverse effects should be reduced, or at least not increased, by the co-administration of two agents

- in order to simplify the treatment, the drug combination should be effective when administered once daily
- the combination should provide better, or at least comparable protection against complications of hypertension compared with individual monotherapies or other therapeutic drug regimens
- the sale price for the combination should be lower, or at least not exceed that of the two components prescribed individually.

There is strong evidence today that all these criteria are met by fixed-dose preparations based on AT$_1$-receptor blockers and HCTZ.[54,55] Fixed low-dose combinations might actually be used as a 'first-line' treatment according to the latest recommendations of the European Society of Hypertension and the European Society of Cardiology.[1] This point of view is shared by the experts of the Joint National Committee in the United States, at least for patients with pre-treatment blood pressures >160/100 mmHg who are most of the time non-responders to monotherapies.[29]

Conclusions

The increased effectiveness obtained by combining an AT$_1$-receptor blocker with another antihypertensive agent, in particular a thiazide diuretic at low dose, is not obtained at the expense of reduced tolerability compared with the individual components administered alone. Fixed-dose combinations containing such agents are therefore likely to become increasingly used not only as second-step therapy but also as first-line treatment choices. The availability of fixed-dose combinations containing AT$_1$-receptor blockers and calcium antagonists might also turn out to be very useful in coming years.

References

1. 2003 European Society of Hypertension–European Society of Cardiology guidelines for the management of arterial hypertension. J Hypertens 2003; 21:1011–53.
2. Marques-Vidal P, Tuomilehto J. Hypertension awareness, treatment and control in the community: is the 'rule of halves' still valid? J Hum Hypertens 1997; 11:213–23.
3. Burt VL, Cutler JA, Higgins M et al. Trends in the prevalence, awareness, treatment, and control of hypertension in the adult US population. Data from the health examination surveys, 1960 to 1991. Hypertension 1995; 26:60–9.
4. Dickerson CJE, Hingorani AD, Ashby MJ, Palmer CR, Brown MJ. Optimisation of antihypertensive treatment by crossover rotation of four major classes. Lancet 1999; 353:2008–13.
5. Brunner HR, Menard J, Waeber B et al. Treating the individual hypertensive patient: considerations on dose, sequential monotherapy and drug combinations. J Hypertens 1990; 8:3–11.
6. Law MR, Moris JK, Jordan RE. Value of low dose combination treatment with blood pressure lowering drugs: analysis of 354 randomized trials. BMJ 2003; 326:1–8.
7. Epstein M, Bakris G. Newer approaches to antihypertensive therapy. Use of fixed-dose combination therapy. Arch Intern Med 1996; 156:1969–78.
8. Waeber B, Brunner HR. Low-dose combinations versus monotherapies in the treatment of hypertension. J Hypertens 1997; 15(Suppl 2):17–20.

9. Ram CV. Antihypertensive efficacy of angiotensin receptor blockers in combination with hydrochlorothiazide: a review of the factorial-design studies. J Clin Hypertens 2004; 6:569–77.
10. Waeber B. Combination therapy with ACE inhibitors/angiotensin II receptor antagonists and diuretics in hypertension. Expert Rev Cardiovasc Ther 2003; 1:43–50.
11. Brunner HR, Waeber B, Nussberger J. Renin secretion responsiveness: understanding the efficacy of renin–angiotensin inhibition. Kidney Int 1988; 26:S80–5.
12. Brunner HR, Gavras H, Laragh JH, Keenan R. Hypertension in man. Explosure of the renin and sodium components using angiotensin II blockade. Circ Res 1974; 34/35(Suppl 1):35–43.
13. Schoenberger JA. Losartan with hydrochlorothiazide in patients with mild to moderate hypertension. J Hypertens 1995; 13(Suppl 1):S43–7.
14. Philip T, Letzel H, Arens HJ. Dose-finding study of candesartan cilexetil plus hydrochlorothiazide in patients with mild to moderate hypertension. J Hum Hypertens 1997; 11(Suppl 2):67–8.
15. Kochar M, Guthrie R, Triscari J, Kassler-Taub K, Reeves RA. Matrix study of irbesartan with hydrochlorothiazide in mild-to-moderate hypertension. Am J Hypertens 1999; 12:797–805.
16. Benz JR, Black HR, Graff A et al. Valsartan and hydrochlorothiazide in patients with essential hypertension. A multiple dose, double-blind, placebo controlled trial comparing combination therapy with monotherapy. J Hum Hypertens 1998; 12:861–6.
17. Chrysant SG, Weber MA, Wang AC, Hinman DJ. Evaluation of antihypertensive therapy with the combination of olmesartan medoxomil and hydrochlorothiazide. Am J Hypertens 2004; 17:252–9.
18. McGill JB, Reilly PA. Telmisartan plus hydrochlorothiazide versus telmisartan or hydrochlorothiazide monotherapy in patients with mild to moderate hypertension: a multicenter, randomized, double-blind, placebo-controlled, parallel-group trial. Clin Ther 2001; 23:833–50.
19. Preston RA, Materson BJ, Reda DJ et al. Age-race subgroup compared with renin profile as predictors of blood pressure response to antihypertensive therapy. Department of Veterans Affairs Cooperative Study Group on Antihypertensive Agents. JAMA 1998; 280:1168–72.
20. Flack JM, Saunders E, Gradman A et al. Antihypertensive efficacy and safety of losartan alone and in combination with hydrochlorothiazide in adult African Americans with mild to moderate hypertension. Clin Ther 2001; 23:1193–208.
21. Plouin PF. Combination therapy with candesartan cilexetil plus hydrochlorothiazide in patients unresponsive to low-dose hydrochlorothiazide. J Hum Hypertens 1997; 11(Suppl 2):65–6.
22. Rosenstock J, Rossi L, Lin CS, MacNeil D, Osbakken M. The effects of irbesartan added to hydrochlorothiazide for the treatment of hypertension in patients non-responsive to hydrochlorothiazide alone. J Clin Pharmacol Ther 1998; 23:433–40.
23. Campbell M, Sonkodi S, Soucek M, Wiecek A. A candesartan cilexetil/hydrochlorothiazide combination tablet provides effective blood pressure control in hypertensive patients inadequately controlled on monotherapy. Clin Exper Hypertens 2001; 23:345–55.
24. Hall D, Motoro R, Littlejohn T et al. Efficacy and tolerability of valsartan in combination with hydrochlorothiazide in essential hypertension. Clin Drug Invest 1998; 16:203–10.
25. Ruilope LM, Malacco E, Khder Y et al. Efficacy and tolerability of combination therapy with valsartan plus hydrochlorothiazide compared with amlodipine monotherapy in hypertensive patients with other cardiovascular risk factors: the VAST study. Clin Ther 2005; 27:578–87.
26. Turnbull F, Neal B, Algert C et al. Effects of different blood pressure-lowering regimens on major cardiovascular events in individuals with and without diabetes mellitus: results of prospectively designed overviews of randomized trials. Arch Intern Med 2005; 165:1410–19.
27. Safar M. Systolic blood pressure, pulse pressure and arterial stiffness as cardiovascular risk factors. Curr Opin Nephrol Hypertens 2001; 10:257–61.
28. Staessen JA, Gasowski J, Wang JG et al. Risks of untreated and treated isolated systolic hypertension in the elderly: meta-analysis of outcome trials. Lancet 2000; 355:865–72.
29. Chobanian AV, Bakris GL, Black HR et al. Seventh report of the Joint National Committee on Prevention, Detection, Evaluation, and Treatment of High Blood Pressure. Hypertension 2003; 42:1206–52.
30. Whitworth JA. 2003 World Health Organization (WHO)/International Society of Hypertension (ISH) statement on management of hypertension. J Hypertens 2003; 21:1983–92.

31. Lemogoum D, Seedat YK, Mabadeje AF et al. Recommendations for prevention, diagnosis and management of hypertension and cardiovascular risk factors in sub-Saharan Africa. J Hypertens 2003; 21:1993–2000.

32. Williams B, Poulter NR, Brown MJ et al. British Hypertension Society guidelines for hypertension management 2004 (BHS-IV): summary. BMJ 2004; 328:634–40.

33. Swales JD. Current clinical practice in hypertension: the EISBERG (Evaluation and Interventions for Systolic Blood pressure Elevation-Regional and Global) project. Am Heart J 1999; 138:231–7.

34. Lloyd-Jones DM, Evans JC, Larson MG, O'Donnell CJ, Levy D. Differential impact of systolic and diastolic blood pressure level on JNC-VI staging. Joint National Committee on Prevention, Detection, Evaluation, and Treatment of High Blood Pressure. Hypertension 1999; 34:381–5.

35. Dahlöf B, Devereux RB, Kjeldsen SE et al. Cardiovascular morbidity and mortality in the Losartan Intervention For Endpoint reduction in hypertension study (LIFE): a randomised trial against atenolol. Lancet 2002; 359:995–1003.

36. Julius S, Kjeldsen SE, Weber M et al. Outcomes in hypertensive patients at high cardiovascular risk treated with regimens based on valsartan or amlodipine: the VALUE randomised trial. Lancet 2004; 363:2022–231.

37. Raskin P, Guthrie R, Flack J, Reeves R, Saini R. The long-term antihypertensive activity and tolerability of irbesartan with hydrochlorothiazide. J Hum Hypertens 1999; 13:683–7.

38. Grassi G, Seravalle G, Dell'Oro R et al. Comparative effects of candesartan and hydrochlorothiazide on blood pressure, insulin sensitivity, and sympathetic drive in obese hypertensive individuals: results of the CROSS study. J Hypertens 2003; 21:1761–9.

39. Jandeleit-Dahm KA, Tikellis C, Reid CM, Johnston CI, Cooper ME. Why blockade of the renin–angiotensin system reduces the incidence of new-onset diabetes. J Hypertens 2005; 23:463–73.

40. Opie LH, Schall R. Old antihypertensives and new diabetes. J Hypertens 2004; 22:1453–8.

41. Kurtz TW, Pravenec M. Antidiabetic mechanisms of angiotensin-converting enzyme inhibitors and angiotensin II receptor antagonists: beyond the renin–angiotensin system. J Hypertens 2004; 22:2253–61.

42. Soffer BA, Wright JT Jr, Pratt JH et al. Effects of losartan on a background of hydrochlorothiazide in patients with hypertension. Hypertension 1995; 26:112–17.

43. Puig JG, Ruilope LM. Uric acid as a cardiovascular risk factor in arterial hypertension. J Hypertens 1999; 17:869–72.

44. Burnier M, Waeber B, Brunner HR. Clinical pharmacology of the angiotensin II receptor antagonist losartan potassium in healthy subjects. J Hum Hypertens 1995; 13(Suppl 1):S23–8.

45. Campbell DJ. The renin–angiotensin and the kallikrein–kinin systems. Int J Biochem Cell Biol 2003; 35:784–91.

46. Tom B, Dendorfer A, Danser AH. Bradykinin, angiotensin-(1-7), and ACE inhibitors: how do they interact? Int J Biochem Cell Biol 2003; 35:792–801.

47. Azizi M, Linhart A, Alexander J et al. Pilot study of combined blockade of the renin–angiotensin system in essential hypertensive patients. J Hypertens 2000; 18:1139–47.

48. Waeber B, Aschwanden R, Sadecky L, Ferber P. Combination of hydrochlorothiazide or benazepril with valsartan in hypertensive patients unresponsive to valsartan alone. J Hypertens 2001; 19:2097–104.

49. Campbell R, Sangalli F, Perticucci E et al. Effects of combined ACE inhibitor and angiotensin II antagonist treatment in human chronic nephropathies. Kidney Int 2003; 63:1094–103.

50. Wolf G, Ritz E. Combination therapy with ACE inhibitors and angiotensin II receptor blockers to halt progression of chronic renal disease: pathophysiology and indications. Kidney Int 2005; 67:799–812.

51. Meredith PA, Elliott HL. Dihydropyridine calcium channel blockers: basic pharmacological similarities but fundamental therapeutic differences. J Hypertens 2004; 22:1641–8.

52. MacGregor GA, Viskoper JR, Antonios TF, He FJ. Efficacy of candesartan cilexetil alone or in combination with amlodipine and hydrochlorothiazide in moderate-to-severe hypertension. UK and Israel Candesartan Investigators. Hypertension 2000; 36:454–60.

53. Andreadis EA, Tsourous GI, Marakomichelakis GE et al. High-dose monotherapy vs low-dose

combination therapy of calcium channel blockers and angiotensin receptor blockers in mild to moderate hypertension. J Hum Hypertens 2005; 19:491–6.

54. Elliott WJ. Is fixed combination therapy appropriate for initial hypertension treatment? Current Hypertens Rep 2002; 4:278–85.

55. Welsh L, Ferro A. Drug treatment of essential hypertension: the case for initial combination therapy. Int J Clin Pract 2004; 58:956–63.

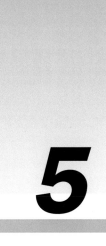

Angiotensin II antagonists in the treatment of patients with renal impairment or failure

Luis Miguel Ruilope and Alejandro de la Sierra

5

Introduction

The kidney plays an important dual role in hypertension and cardiovascular diseases, both contributing to the increase in systemic blood pressure and being damaged by its long-term consequences.[1] Chronic renal disease is characterized by a gradual loss of renal function and an increased cardiovascular risk.[2] A disturbed renal function per se is a major predictor of cardiovascular complications.[3] In patients with end-stage renal disease, the risk of cardiovascular-related death is as much as 3–20 times greater than in healthy subjects and is associated with a high incidence of myocardial infarction, left ventricular hypertrophy, and congestive heart failure.[3,4] Renal function per se is a powerful predictor of cardiovascular outcome in patients with hypertension or heart failure in the absence of primary renal disease,[5–10] and even minor increases in serum creatinine above normal values correlate strongly with future cardiovascular morbidity.

The recognition that cardiovascular, cerebrovascular, and renal disease processes are interrelated has important consequences for treatment. Any strategies aimed at preventing disease must consider the system as an integrated whole and assign equal importance to the preservation of kidney function and the lowering of blood pressure.

During the past decades, a tremendous body of research, both experimental and clinical, has unequivocally shown that pharmacologic blockade of the renin–angiotensin system (RAS) with angiotensin converting enzyme inhibitors

Table 5.1
Main clinical trials with angiotensin II receptor blockers (ARBs) in patients with renal disease.

Study	Disease	ARB	Comparative drug
ARBs vs conventional therapy			
IRMA-2	Type 2 DM + early nephropathy	Irbesartan	Placebo
MARVAL	Type 2 DM + early nephropathy	Valsartan	Amlodipine
IDNT	Type 2 DM + overt nephropathy	Irbesartan	Placebo or amlodipine
RENAAL	Type 2 DM + overt nephropathy	Losartan	Placebo
ARBs vs ACE inhibitors or ARBs + ACE inhibitors			
DETAIL	Type 2 DM + early nephropathy	Telmisartan	Enalapril
COOPERATE	Non-DM overt nephropathy	Losartan + trandolapril	Losartan or trandolapril
CALM	Type 2 DM + early nephropathy	Candesartan + lisinopril	Candesartan or lisinopril

DM = diabetes mellitus.

(ACEIs) or angiotensin receptor blockers (ARBs) slows progressive renal function loss more effectively than other antihypertensive treatments.[11]

In the first edition of this book we presented experimental data suggesting that ARBs could be a valid alternative to ACEI in the treatment of diabetic hypertensives and patients with renal impairment.[12] Now, 6 years later, these experimental data have been corroborated by a considerable amount of clinical trials demonstrating the beneficial effects of ARBs in such patients (Table 5.1).

Mild renal dysfunction in the general population

Mild renal dysfunction, defined as a glomerular filtration rate (GFR) $<60\,ml/min/1.73\,m^2$ and/or the presence of microalbuminuria $>30\,mg/24\,h$ is associated with a significantly increased risk of cardiovascular disease and death.[13–15] Mild renal abnormalities are present in around 10% of the general population, and the risk of total and cardiovascular mortality, stroke, and heart failure is considerably increased in these individuals (Figure 5.1). Moreover, the recent European Prospective Investigation into Cancer in Norfolk (EPIC-Norfolk) study followed prospectively a population-based cohort of over 23 000 individuals in a general British population aged between 40 and 79 years for 7 years.[16] Rates of cardiovascular disease-related death and all-cause mortality correlated significantly with increasing levels of albuminuria, even at values lying within the range of 'normoalbuminuria' (Figure 5.2). Microalbuminuria was present in 12% of this unselected population and independently predicted a 30% increased risk of cardiovascular disease and a 50% increased risk of stroke.[17,18] Similarly, in a Danish population-based study, mild renal dysfunction predicted higher cardiovascular mortality, which

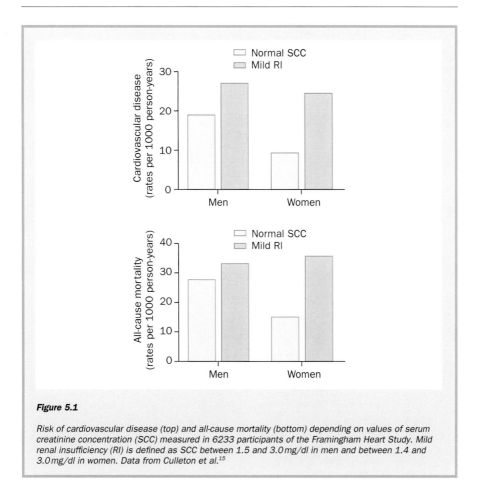

Figure 5.1

Risk of cardiovascular disease (top) and all-cause mortality (bottom) depending on values of serum creatinine concentration (SCC) measured in 6233 participants of the Framingham Heart Study. Mild renal insufficiency (RI) is defined as SCC between 1.5 and 3.0 mg/dl in men and between 1.4 and 3.0 mg/dl in women. Data from Culleton et al.[15]

increased by 11% for every 5 μmol/L increase in serum creatinine concentrations and by 26% for every 5 ml/min/1.73 m^2 decrease in GFR.[19]

Mild renal dysfunction in hypertension

In hypertensive patients, mild renal dysfunction ranges from 10% to 40% in high-risk populations,[8,20] and also impairs cardiovascular prognosis.[15,21] In fact, serum creatinine concentrations have been found to closely correlate with increased cardiovascular risk. For example, the Heart Outcomes Prevention Evaluation (HOPE)[8] and the Hypertension Optimal Treatment (HOT)[10] studies found a twofold higher incidence of cardiovascular events with mildly elevated serum creatinine concentrations (≥1.4 mg/dl; 123 μmol/L) in people at high cardiovascular risk due to coronary artery disease and/or hypertension. In the Hypertension Detection and Follow-up Program (HDFP),[21] a fivefold difference in cardiovascular mortality

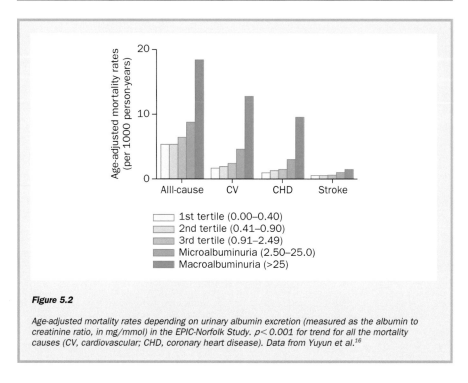

Figure 5.2

Age-adjusted mortality rates depending on urinary albumin excretion (measured as the albumin to creatinine ratio, in mg/mmol) in the EPIC-Norfolk Study. p< 0.001 for trend for all the mortality causes (CV, cardiovascular; CHD, coronary heart disease). Data from Yuyun et al.[16]

rates was found between patients in the lowest quintile of serum creatinine levels and those in the highest, whereas the International Nifedipine GITS study: Intervention as a Goal in Hypertension Treatment (INSIGHT)[6] found that, of all the risk factors evaluated, the presence of proteinuria ($\geq$0.5 g/24 h) predicted the highest risk of a cardiovascular event or death in patients with hypertension.

Therapeutic strategies to protect renal function

The natural history of renal impairment mirrors that of cardiovascular disease (Figure 5.3), and the two pathologies share many risk factors, as well as similar stages of progression. Given that renal damage and cardiovascular disease go hand in hand, therapeutic approaches to preventing or reducing renal disease must consider both the control of blood pressure and the preservation of renal function.

Tight control of blood pressure is essential to reduce cardiovascular risk and to impede the progression of renal disease.[22] International guidelines have established that goal blood pressure in the presence of renal failure should be <130/80 mmHg, or even lower (<125/75 mmHg) in the presence of overt proteinuria (>1 g/24 h).[23–25]

Lowering blood pressure via angiotensin II blockade, using either an ACEI or an ARB, appears to confer better protection against hypertensive renal damage than blood pressure lowering by

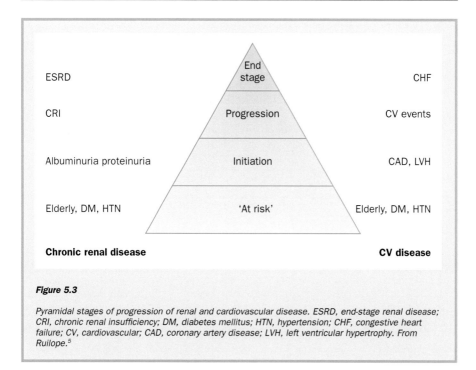

Figure 5.3

Pyramidal stages of progression of renal and cardiovascular disease. ESRD, end-stage renal disease; CRI, chronic renal insufficiency; DM, diabetes mellitus; HTN, hypertension; CHF, congestive heart failure; CV, cardiovascular; CAD, coronary artery disease; LVH, left ventricular hypertrophy. From Ruilope.[5]

other mechanisms. Angiotensin II, the principal peptide of the RAS, coordinates many of the pathologic processes involved in the development of hypertension, and cardiovascular and renal disease. The discovery that the kidney has its own local RAS that is activated independently under hyperglycemic conditions highlights the importance of this peptide in renal physiology and pathology, especially in patients with diabetes.[26,27]

Clinical data suggest that ARBs help to preserve the intrinsic renal autoregulatory mechanisms and enhance renal vasodilation. In arterial hypertension, GFR autoregulation is often impaired or absent, allowing the transmission of systemic blood pressure directly to the glomeruli.[28–30] Some antihypertensives, for example calcium channel blockers, can seriously impede GFR autoregulation in such a way that serum creatinine levels actually rise as blood pressure falls.[28] In contrast, ARBs appear to be able to reduce blood pressure while preserving endogenous renal autoregulation.[31]

ARBs may also improve renal vasodilation and renal plasma flow. Studies in healthy volunteers have demonstrated that moderate induced hyperglycemia activates an intrarenal RAS system, leading to enhanced renal vasodilation and greater renal plasma flow.[26,27] The activation of the intrarenal RAS enhances the renal response to ARBs; in healthy adults on a high-sodium diet, induced hyperglycemia produced a 12% increase in renal plasma flow, whereas the administration of eprosartan increased renal plasma flow by a further 14% without affecting GFR.[27] Under normoglycemic conditions, the ARB had no effect on renal plasma flow or GFR, and plasma renin and plasma angiotensin II levels remained unchanged.

Antiproteinuric effects of the ARBs

Proteinuria is an important marker of glomerular damage and promotes the progression of renal lesions; it also represents a powerful predictor of the long-term beneficial effect of antihypertensive therapy.[32–34] Several studies[35–41] have shown that ARBs consistently reduce urinary albumin concentration in patients with type 2 diabetes, in patients with non-diabetic nephropathy, in renal transplant recipients, and in experimental models.

Recently, Zandbergen et al[40] demonstrated the antiproteinuric effects of losartan in normotensive patients with type 2 diabetes and persistent microalbuminuria. Using a randomized, double-blind, placebo-controlled study protocol, these investigators showed that patients receiving 50 mg losartan over the initial 5 weeks of the study demonstrated a 25% reduction in urinary albumin excretion (UAE) vs 6.8% in the placebo group. This value increased to a 34% reduction vs an increase of 1.3% in the placebo group after a dose of 100 mg over the subsequent 5 weeks. The adjusted mean difference in UAE rate between losartan and placebo at 5 weeks was $-16.9\,\mu g/min$ ($p < 0.001$). A multivariate analysis showed that the alterations in UAE occurred independently of blood pressure, suggesting an independent renoprotective effect of losartan.

In type 2 diabetic patients two well-controlled, randomized trials, the Irbesartan in Patients with type 2 diabetes and Microalbuminuria (IRMA-2)[42] and the MicroAlbuminuria Reduction with VALsartan (MARVAL)[43] trial have both demonstrated that ARBs reduce the progression from microalbuminuria to overt nephropathy.

The IRMA-2 study

IRMA-2[42] was a multinational, randomized, double-blind study involving 590 patients (~70% male and 97% white) with type 2 diabetes and hypertension. It showed that patients receiving irbesartan (150 mg or 300 mg) had a reduced rate of progression of microalbuminuria (UAE rate = 20–200 $\mu g/min$ in two of three overnight urine collections) to clinical proteinuria.

Approximately 5.3% of patients receiving 300 mg irbesartan, 9.7% of patients receiving 150 mg irbesartan, and 14.9% of placebo-treated patients reached the primary end point (time to onset of diabetic nephropathy). By 2 years, restoration to normoalbuminuria ($<20\,\mu g/min$) occurred in 34% of patients in the irbesartan 300 mg group ($p < 0.006$ vs placebo), 24% in the irbesartan 150 mg group, and 21% in the placebo group (Figure 5.4). The effects of irbesartan were independent of alterations in systemic blood pressure.

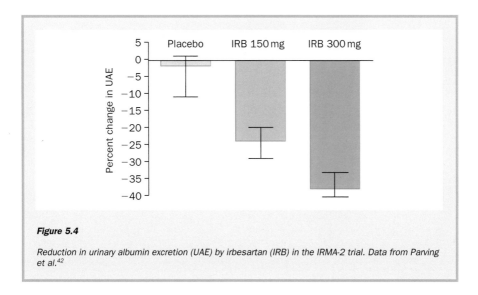

Figure 5.4

Reduction in urinary albumin excretion (UAE) by irbesartan (IRB) in the IRMA-2 trial. Data from Parving et al.[42]

The MARVAL trial

The MARVAL trial[43] was a randomized study that assessed the effects of valsartan or amlodipine on urinary albumin excretion in 322 patients with type 2 diabetes and microalbuminuria, with or without hypertension. Subjects were predominantly male (80%) and white (87%), with an age range of 35–75 years. A diuretic (bendrofluazide) or α-blocker (doxazosin) was added to valsartan or amlodipine treatment as needed to control blood pressure (target = 135/85 mmHg). A total of 291 patients completed the study (valsartan, $n = 146$; amlodipine, $n = 145$). More patients receiving valsartan (29.9%) than amlodipine (14.5%) achieved normoalbuminuria at week 24 (between-treatment difference = 15.4%; $p < 0.001$) despite similar reductions in blood pressure. Mean albumin excretion rates decreased from 58 to 32 μg/min in valsartan-treated patients and from 55 to 51 μg/min in amlodipine-treated patients ($p < 0.001$).

Impact of ARBs on renal and cardiovascular outcomes in type 2 DM with proteinuria

Over the past decade, the advent of evidence-based medicine has generated demand for outcome data from large clinical trials, which are currently considered the most valid measure of clinical efficacy. Hard end points such as mortality or morbidity are needed not only to properly position new and old treatments in a constantly changing therapeutic armamentarium but also to help make decisions about the cost-effectiveness of various interventions.

Two long-term end point studies in patients with type 2 diabetes and nephropathy have addressed whether the marked antiproteinuric effect of ARBs translates into improved renal

Table 5.2
Relative risks (95% CIs) for different renal end points in the two outcome trials with angiotensin receptor blockers in patients with type 2 diabees and overt nephropathy.

End point	RENAAL (LOS vs PCBO)	IDNT (IRB vs PCBO)	IDNT (IRB vs AML)
Primary end point	0.84 (0.72–0.98)	0.80 (0.66–0.97)	0.77 (0.63–0.93)
Doubling of SC	0.75 (0.61–0.92)	0.67 (0.52–0.87)	0.63 (0.48–0.81)
ESRD	0.72 (0.58–0.89)	0.77 (0.57–1.03)	0.77 (0.57–1.03)
Death	1.02 (0.81–1.27)	0.92 (0.69–1.23)	1.04 (0.77–1.40)

LOS, losartan; PCBO, placebo; IRB, irbesartan; AML, amlodipine; SC, serum creatinine; ESRD, end-stage renal disease.

outcomes. These studies are RENAAL[44] and IDNT.[45] Both trials involved similar study populations: mainly hypertensive patients with type 2 diabetes with mild to moderate renal failure (serum creatinine concentration between 1.0 and 3.0 mg/dl) and overt proteinuria. The results of outcome studies such as these provide important evidence-based guidance for physicians and have resulted in a marked change in the treatment paradigm of patients with type 2 diabetic nephropathy (Table 5.2).

The RENAAL Study

The RENAAL study[44] assessed the potential renoprotective benefits of specific AII blockade with losartan in terms of end-stage renal disease or death. It was a multinational, double-blind, placebo-controlled trial that investigated whether losartan, either alone or in combination with conventional antihypertensive therapy, reduced the number of patients with type 2 diabetes who experienced a doubling of serum creatinine, end-stage renal disease, or death compared with placebo-treated patients. In addition, the study assessed the effects of losartan on cardiovascular mortality, morbidity, and proteinuria as well as on quality of life and healthcare resource utilization.

A total of 1513 patients with type 2 diabetes, either hypertensive or normotensive, were randomly assigned to receive losartan (50–100 mg/day) or placebo, in addition to their existing antihypertensive therapy for 4 years. Patients had severe renal disease with macroalbuminuria and serum creatinine between 1.3 and 3.0 mg/dl, and were all likely to progress to dialysis. The study population comprised male (63%) and female (37%) patients who were white (49%), black (15%), Asian (17%), Hispanic (18%), or another race (1%), and had a mean age of 60 years. Patients received conventional antihypertensive treatment (i.e. calcium channel blockers, diuretics, α-blockers, β-blockers, and centrally acting agents) as needed to control blood pressure.

Patients receiving losartan demonstrated renal protection over a follow-up period of 3.4 years. Compared with placebo-treated patients, patients receiving losartan demonstrated a 16% reduction ($p = 0.02$) in the primary composite end point (doubling of serum creatinine, end-stage renal disease, or death from any cause), a 25% risk reduction for doubling of creatinine ($p = 0.006$), a 28% reduction in the risk of end-stage renal disease ($p = 0.002$), and a 20% risk reduction in the composite end point of end-stage renal disease and death ($p = 0.01$). Patients receiving losartan also demonstrated a 35% decrease in the level of proteinuria, as evidenced by a significant decrease in the urinary albumin/creatinine ratio ($p < 0.001$). No differences were observed for the composite end point of cardiovascular morbidity or mortality, although losartan was associated with a 32% reduction in the risk of hospitalization for heart failure ($p = 0.005$).

The renoprotective benefits of losartan occurred over and above the effects on blood pressure control (the losartan and placebo groups had similar trough systolic and diastolic blood pressures during the study) and the effects of other therapies including aspirin, β-blockers, and lipid-lowering agents. Losartan plus conventional antihypertensive therapy demonstrated excellent tolerability, similar to that in the placebo group. Similar numbers of patients in the two study groups discontinued because of adverse events.

The IDNT

IDNT,[45] a prospective, randomized, double-blind, placebo-controlled clinical trial, assessed whether the ARB irbesartan or the calcium channel blocker amlodipine protected against the progression of nephropathy in patients with type 2 diabetes. The study involved 1715 diabetic hypertensive patients with proteinuria (defined as urinary albumin excretion >900 mg/day) and serum creatinine between 1.0 and 3.0 mg/dL in women and between 1.2 and 3.0 mg/dl in men. The study population comprised men (66%) and women (34%) who were predominantly white (72%), with a mean age of 59 years. Patients received either irbesartan (300 mg/day) or amlodipine (10 mg/day) for a mean duration of 2.6 years to achieve a target blood pressure of 135/85 mmHg. The primary end point of the study was a composite of the time to a doubling of the baseline serum creatinine, development of end-stage renal disease, or death.

Irbesartan-treated patients generally demonstrated better renal outcomes than those in the amlodipine group. These included a 20% lower risk ($p = 0.02$) for the primary end point than in the placebo group (23% lower risk vs the amlodipine group; $p = 0.006$), a 33% lower risk ($p = 0.003$) of doubling of serum creatinine than in the placebo group (37% lower risk vs the amlodipine group; $p < 0.001$), and a 23% lower relative risk of end-stage renal disease than in either the placebo or amlodipine groups (not significant for either comparison). Serum creatinine increased 24% more slowly in the irbesartan group than in the placebo group ($p = 0.008$) and 21% more slowly than in the amlodipine group ($p = 0.02$). However, no differences were found between groups with respect to the secondary composite end point of cardiovascular events, including cardiovascular death, myocardial infarction, hospitalization for heart failure, or stroke. Irbesartan provided overall benefits even though both groups had comparable degrees of blood pressure control.

Factors that can maximize the renoprotective effects of ARBs; ARBs used in combination

Studies published to date suggest that using ARBs in combination with other antihypertensives affords substantially better renoprotection. The benefit of using ARBs in this way was clearly demonstrated in the RENAAL study.[44] Losartan 50–100 mg was given against a background of conventional antihypertensive therapy that included diuretics, calcium channel blockers, α-blockers, β-blockers, and centrally acting agents. The combination of an ARB plus other antihypertensives proved more effective than either therapy alone.

Preliminary studies using ARBs in combination with ACE inhibitors to provide more complete angiotensin II blockade have shown that this combination is a powerful one, resulting in even greater reductions in proteinuria and slowing of renal impairment (Figure 5.5). In a recent pilot

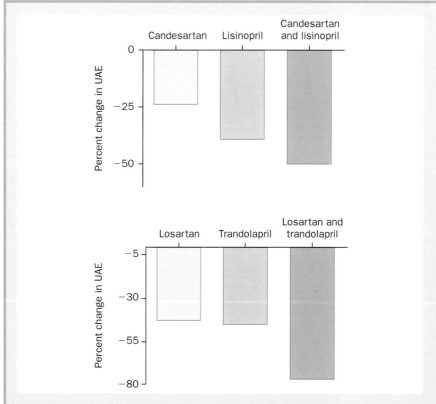

Figure 5.5

Reduction in urinary albumin excretion (UAE) by ACE inhibitors, angiotensin II receptor blockers or the combination of both in two studies in patients with type 2 diabetes and microalbuminuria (CALM; top) or non-diabetic nephropathy (COOPERATE, bottom). Data from Mogensen et al[54] and Nakao et al.[53]

study, Segura and colleagues[46] evaluated the maximum recommended doses of valsartan 160 mg and benazepril 20 mg, alone or in combination, in 36 patients with hypertension (>140/90 mmHg) and primary renal disease (proteinuria >1.5 g/24 h). After 6 months of treatment, reductions in blood pressure and serum creatinine concentrations were equivalent in all treatment arms but the combination produced a significant additive reduction ($p < 0.05$) in proteinuria compared with baseline values. Similar benefits have been found in other small-scale studies in both diabetic and non-diabetic renal disease patients using high-dose combinations of different ARBs and ACE inhibitors: valsartan and benazepril,[47–49] losartan and lisinopril,[50] irbesartan and enalapril,[51] and irbesartan and fosinopril.[52]

These promising results have been reproduced in two large-scale, prospective studies, the combination treatment of angiotensin II receptor blocker and angiotensin converting enzyme inhibitor in non-diabetic renal disease (COOPERATE)[53] and the Candesartan And Lisinopril effect on Microalbuminuria (CALM) study.[54] In the 3-year COOPERATE study, conducted on 336 patients with non-diabetic renal disease and proteinuria, the combination of an ACE inhibitor (trandolapril 3 mg) and an ARB (losartan 100 mg) halved the proportion of patients reaching the primary composite end point of the doubling of the serum creatinine concentration or the need to enter dialysis (11%), compared with either treatment alone (23% for both trandolapril and losartan) ($p = 0.02$). This beneficial effect was despite similar reductions in blood pressure with monotherapy and combination therapy. Importantly, this trial demonstrated that there is a plateau of effect for ACE inhibition on renoprotection: during the run-in phase, the authors uptitrated the ACE inhibitor to 6 mg while monitoring proteinuria, and identified a leveling-off effect at 3 mg, the maximum effective dose for lowering proteinuria.

In CALM,[54] which was a 6-month study conducted on 199 patients with type 2 diabetes, hypertension, and microalbuminuria, a combination of candesartan 16 mg and lisinopril 20 mg was significantly more effective in reducing the albumin:creatinine ratio (50% reduction; 95% CI = 36–61; $p < 0.001$) than candesartan (24% reduction; 95% CI = 0–43; $p = 0.05$) or lisinopril (39% reduction, 95% CI = 20–54; $p < 0.001$) alone.

ARBs compared to ACE inhibitors in patients with renal disease

The two aforementioned studies (COOPERATE[53] and CALM[54]) provide some indirect evidence of the comparative renoprotective effect between ARBs and ACE inhibitors. As stated, in the COOPERATE trial[53] the reduction of the primary composite end point was the same in patients treated with trandolapril or losartan. In the CALM trial,[54] the antiproteinuric effect of lisinopril was somewhat greater than that observed with candesartan. These two studies were not specifically designed to demonstrate differences between the two drug classes.

The Diabetics Exposed to Telmisartan and Enalapril Study Group (DETAIL)[55] examined the renoprotective effect of telmisartan 80 mg vs enalapril 20 mg in 250 diabetics with early nephropathy. The primary end point was the change in GFR (measurement of plasma clearance of iohexol). At the end of the follow-up (5 years), GFR decreased 17.9 ml/min/1.73 m^2 in the telmisartan group and 14.9 ml/min/1.73 m^2 in enalapril-treated patients. As the study was planned as a non-inferiority trial, the statistical analysis revealed that telmisartan was not inferior to enalapril in renoprotection.

Closing remarks

Renal function is an intrinsic component of the cardiovascular continuum and a major risk factor for cardiovascular morbidity and mortality. Even mild renal impairment greatly increases the risk of cardiovascular events, and so therapeutic strategies must encompass control of renal function, as well as control of blood pressure.

Blood pressure reduction alone is sufficient to improve renal function in patients with advanced nephropathy and high blood pressure, but in less-impaired patients angiotensin II blockade provides superior renoprotection. ARBs dramatically impede the progression to overt nephropathy in patients with evidence of primary renal disease and can reverse early indications of renal impairment in patients with mild renal abnormalities. Greater protection can be afforded by uptitrating the ARBs to the highest effective dose, but using ARBs and ACE inhibitors together promises to provide greater renoprotection.

References

1. Ruilope LM, Campo C, Rodriguez-Artalejo F et al. Blood pressure and renal function: therapeutic implications. J Hypertens 1996; 14:1259–63.
2. Baigent C, Burbury K, Wheeler D. Premature cardiovascular disease in chronic renal failure. Lancet 2000; 356:147–52.
3. Ruilope LM, van Veldhuisen DJ, Ritz E, Luscher TF. Renal function: the Cinderella of cardiovascular risk profile. J Am Coll Cardiol 2001; 38:1782–7.
4. Rostand SG, Brunzell JD, Cannon RO, Victor RG. Cardiovascular complications in renal failure. J Am Soc Nephrol 1991; 2:1053–62.
5. Ruilope LM. Renin–angiotensin–aldosterone system blockade and renal protection: angiotensin-converting enzyme inhibitors or angiotensin II receptor blockers? Acta Diabetol 2005; 42(Suppl 1):S33–41.
6. Brown MJ, Palmer CR, Castaigne A et al. Morbidity and mortality in patients randomised to double-blind treatment with a long-acting calcium-channel blocker or diuretic in the International Nifedipine GITS study: Intervention as a Goal in Hypertension Treatment (INSIGHT). Lancet 2000; 356:366–72.
7. Hillege HL, Girbes AR, de Kam PJ et al. Renal function, neurohormonal activation, and survival in patients with chronic heart failure. Circulation 2000; 102:203–10.
8. Mann JF, Gerstein HC, Pogue J, Bosch J, Yusuf S. Renal insufficiency as a predictor of cardiovascular outcomes and the impact of ramipril: the HOPE randomized trial. Ann Intern Med 2001; 134:629–36.
9. Dries DL, Exner DV, Domanski MJ, Greenberg B, Stevenson LW. The prognostic implications of renal insufficiency in asymptomatic and symptomatic patients with left ventricular systolic dysfunction. J Am Coll Cardiol 2000; 35:681–9.
10. Ruilope LM, Salvetti A, Jamerson K et al. Renal function and intensive lowering of blood pressure in

hypertensive participants of the hypertension optimal treatment (HOT) study. J Am Soc Nephrol 2001; 12:218–25.

11. Remuzzi G, Ruggenenti P, Perico N. Chronic renal diseases: renoprotective benefits of renin–angiotensin system inhibition. Ann Intern Med 2002; 136:604–15.

12. Ruilope LM, de la Sierra A. Angiotensin II receptor antagonists in diabetic hypertensives and hypertensives with renal impairment. In: Mancia G, ed. Angiotensin II receptor antagonists in perspective. London: Martin Dunitz; 2000: 91–105.

13. Leoncini G, Viazzi F, Parodi D et al. Mild renal dysfunction and subclinical cardiovascular damage in primary hypertension. Hypertension 2003; 42:14–18.

14. Mann JF, Gerstein HC, Dulau-Florea I, Lonn E. Cardiovascular risk in patients with mild renal insufficiency. Kidney Int 2003; 63(Suppl 84):S192–6.

15. Culleton BF, Larson MG, Wilson PW et al. Cardiovascular disease and mortality in a community-based cohort with mild renal insufficiency. Kidney Int 1999; 56:2214–19.

16. Yuyun MF, Khaw KT, Luben R et al. Microalbuminuria independently predicts all-cause and cardiovascular mortality in a British population: the European Prospective Investigation into Cancer in Norfolk (EPIC-Norfolk) population study. Int J Epidemiol 2004; 33:189–98.

17. Yuyun MF, Khaw KT, Luben R et al. Microalbuminuria, cardiovascular risk factors and cardiovascular morbidity in a British population: the EPIC-Norfolk population-based study. Eur J Cardiovasc Prev Rehabil 2004; 11:207–13.

18. Yuyun MF, Khaw KT, Luben R et al. Microalbuminuria and stroke in a British population: the European Prospective Investigation into Cancer in Norfolk (EPIC-Norfolk) population study. J Intern Med 2004; 255:247–56.

19. Henry RM, Kostense PJ, Bos G et al. Mild renal insufficiency is associated with increased cardiovascular mortality: the Hoorn Study. Kidney Int 2002; 62:1402–7.

20. Pontremoli R, Sofia A, Ravera M et al. Prevalence and clinical correlates of microalbuminuria in essential hypertension: the MAGIC Study. Microalbuminuria: A Genoa Investigation on Complications. Hypertension 1997; 30:1135–43.

21. Shulman NB, Ford CE, Hall WD et al. Prognostic value of serum creatinine and effect of treatment of hypertension on renal function. Results from the hypertension detection and follow-up program. Hypertension 1989; 13(Suppl):I80–93.

22. Ruilope LM, Campo C, Rodicio JL. Blood pressure control, proteinuria and renal outcome in chronic renal failure. Curr Opin Nephrol Hypertens 1998; 7:145–8.

23. Chobanian AV, Bakris GL, Black HR et al. The Seventh Report of the Joint National Committee on Prevention, Detection, Evaluation, and Treatment of High Blood Pressure: The JNC 7 Report. JAMA 2003; 289:2560–72.

24. Guidelines Committee. 2003 European Society of Hypertension–European Society of Cardiology guidelines for the management of arterial hypertension. J Hypertens 2003; 21:1011–53.

25. National Kidney Foundation. K-DOQI clinical practice guidelines on hypertension and antihypertensive agents in chronic kidney disease. Am J Kidney Dis 2004; 43:S1–290.

26. Osei SY, Price DA, Fisher ND et al. Hyperglycemia and angiotensin mediated control of the renal circulation in healthy humans. Hypertension 1999; 33:559–64.

27. Osei SY, Price DA, Laffel LM, Lansang MC, Hollenberg NK. Effect of angiotensin II antagonist eprosartan on hyperglycemia-induced activation of intrarenal renin angiotensin system in healthy humans. Hypertension 2000; 36:122–6.

28. Christensen PK, Akram K, Konig KB, Parving HH. Autoregulation of glomerular filtration rate in patients with type 2 diabetes during isradipine therapy. Diabetes Care 2003; 26:156–62.

29. Parving HH, Kastrup H, Smidt UM et al. Impaired autoregulation of glomerular filtration rate in type 1 (insulin-dependent) diabetic patients with nephropathy. Diabetologia 1984; 27:547–52.

30. Segura J, Christiansen H, Campo C, Ruilope LM. How to titrate ACE inhibitors and angiotensin receptor blockers in renal patients: according to blood pressure or proteinuria? Curr Hypertens Rep 2003; 5:426–9.

31. Christensen PK, Lund S, Parving HH. Autoregulated glomerular filtration rate during candesartan treatment in hypertensive type 2 diabetic patients. Kidney Int 2001; 60:1435–42.

32. De Jong PE, Navis G, de Zeeuw D. Renoprotective therapy: titration against urinary protein excretion. Lancet 1999; 354:352–3.

33. Nelson RG, Bennett PH, Beck GJ et al. Development and progression of renal disease in Pima Indians with non-insulin-dependent diabetes mellitus. N Engl J Med 1996; 335:1636–42.

34. Rossing P, Hommel E, Smidt UM, Parving HH. Reduction in albuminuria predicts a beneficial effect on diminishing the progression of human diabetic nephropathy during antihypertensive treatment. Diabetologia 1994; 37:511–16.

35. Gansevoort RT, de Zeeuw D, de Jong PE. Is the antiproteinuric effect of ACE inhibition mediated by interference in the renin–angiotensin system? Kidney Int 1994; 45:861–7.

36. Kohzuki M, Yasujima M, Kanazawa M et al. Antihypertensive and renal-protective effects of losartan in streptozotocin diabetic rats. J Hypertens 1995; 13:97–103.

37. Lacourciere Y, Belanger A, Godin C et al. Long-term comparison of losartan and enalapril on kidney function in hypertensive type 2 diabetics with early nephropathy. Kidney Int 2000; 58:762–9.

38. Lafayette RA, Mayer G, Park SK, Meyer TW. Angiotensin II receptor blockade limits glomerular injury in rats with reduced renal mass. J Clin Invest 1992; 90:766–71.

39. Pollock DM, Divish BJ, Polakowski JS, Opgenorth TJ. Angiotensin II receptor blockade improves renal function in rats with reduced renal mass. J Pharmacol Exp Ther 1993; 267:657–63.

40. Zandbergen AA, Baggen MG, Lamberts SW et al. Effect of losartan on microalbuminuria in normotensive patients with type 2 diabetes mellitus. A randomized clinical trial. Ann Intern Med 2003; 139:90–6.

41. Andersen S, Rossing P, Juhl TR et al. Optimal dose of losartan for renoprotection in diabetic nephropathy. Nephrol Dial Transplant 2002; 17:1413–18.

42. Parving HH, Lehnert H, Bröchner-Mortensen J et al. The effect of irbesartan on the development of diabetic nephropathy in patients with type 2 diabetes. N Engl J Med 2001; 345:870–8.

43. Viberti G, Wheeldon NM. Microalbuminuria reduction with valsartan in patients with type 2 diabetes mellitus: a blood pressure-independent effect. Circulation 2002; 106:672–8.

44. Brenner BM, Cooper ME, de Zeeuw D et al. Effects of losartan on renal and cardiovascular outcomes in patients with type 2 diabetes and nephropathy. N Engl J Med 2001; 345:861–9.

45. Lewis EJ, Hunsicker LG, Clarke WR et al. Renoprotective effect of the angiotensin-receptor antagonist irbesartan in patients with nephropathy due to type 2 diabetes. N Engl J Med 2001; 345:851–60.

46. Segura J, Praga M, Campo C, Rodicio JL, Ruilope LM. Combination is better than monotherapy with ACE inhibitor or angiotensin receptor antagonist at recommended doses. J Renin Angiotensin Aldosterone Syst 2003; 4:43–7.

47. Campbell R, Sangalli F, Perticucci E et al. Effects of combined ACE inhibitor and angiotensin II antagonist treatment in human chronic nephropathies. Kidney Int 2003; 63:1094–103.

48. Jacobsen P, Andersen S, Jensen BR, Parving HH. Additive effect of ACE inhibition and angiotensin II receptor blockade in type I diabetic patients with diabetic nephropathy. J Am Soc Nephrol 2003; 14:992–9.

49. Ruilope LM, Aldigier JC, Ponticelli C et al. Safety of the combination of valsartan and benazepril in patients with chronic renal disease. European Group for the Investigation of Valsartan in Chronic Renal Disease. J Hypertens 2000; 18:89–95.

50. Laverman GD, Navis G, Henning RH, de Jong PE, de Zeeuw D. Dual renin–angiotensin system blockade at optimal doses for proteinuria. Kidney Int 2002; 62:1020–5.

51. Jacobsen P, Andersen S, Rossing K, Jensen BR, Parving HH. Dual blockade of the renin–angiotensin system versus maximal recommended dose of ACE inhibition in diabetic nephropathy. Kidney Int 2003; 63:1874–80.

52. Ferrari P, Marti HP, Pfister M, Frey FJ. Additive antiproteinuric effect of combined ACE inhibition and angiotensin II receptor blockade. J Hypertens 2002; 20:125–30.

53. Nakao N, Yoshimura A, Morita H et al. Combination treatment of angiotensin-II receptor blocker and angiotensin-converting-enzyme inhibitor in non-diabetic renal disease (COOPERATE): a randomised controlled trial. Lancet 2003; 361:117–24.

54. Mogensen CE, Neldam S, Tikkanen I et al. Randomised controlled trial of dual blockade of

renin–angiotensin system in patients with hypertension, microalbuminuria, and non-insulin dependent diabetes: the candesartan and lisinopril microalbuminuria (CALM) study. BMJ 2000; 321:1440–4.

55. Barnett AH, Bain SC, Bouter P et al. Angiotensin-receptor blockade versus converting-enzyme inhibition in type 2 diabetes and nephropathy. N Engl J Med 2004; 351:1952–61.

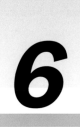

The antidiabetic effect of angiotensin II receptor antagonists: evidence, mechanisms, and clinical significance

Theodore W Kurtz

Introduction

Epidemiologic studies have indicated that the risk for diabetes in untreated patients with hypertension is approximately 2–2.5 times greater than in normotensive subjects.[1] Although the benefits of hypertension control on cardiovascular morbidity and mortality are widely recognized, the effects of antihypertensive drugs on the risk for diabetes are less well understood. Recent studies have suggested that the risk for diabetes in patients treated with angiotensin converting enzyme (ACE) inhibitors or angiotensin receptor blockers (ARBs) is lower than in those treated with other antihypertensive drugs.[2–6] For example, Opie and Schall have estimated that treating 60–70 hypertensive patients for 4 years with a modern agent such as an ARB or an ACE inhibitor instead of a diuretic or β-blocker would avoid one new case of diabetes.[7] Hypertension is also known to frequently occur as part of a complex metabolic syndrome characterized by the clustering of multiple risk factors for both cardiovascular disease and diabetes. The metabolic syndrome is associated with a two- to fourfold increased risk for cardiovascular mortality and a five- to ninefold increased risk for diabetes.[8–10] Thus, the availability of antihypertensive drugs with antidiabetic properties could be of particular value in patients with hypertension and the metabolic syndrome. Accordingly, there is growing interest in the possibility that at least some drugs that interfere with the renin–angiotensin system may have the capacity to increase insulin sensitivity and decrease the risk of type 2 diabetes. Here we review the clinical evidence, mechanisms, and clinical significance of the antidiabetic effects of angiotensin II receptor blockers. The primary focus will be on antidiabetic effects for the prevention of diabetes rather than for amelioration of existing diabetes.

Evidence

Randomized, placebo-controlled clinical trials that are prospectively designed to focus on new-onset diabetes as a major end point are required to assess the true antidiabetic potential of different ARBs. To date, such definitive trial results have not been reported and, therefore, it is not yet possible to draw firm conclusions regarding the antidiabetic effects of ARBs in general or about any ARB in particular. Nevertheless, a considerable amount of indirect clinical and experimental evidence has accumulated that strongly suggests potential antidiabetic effects for at least some of the ARBs in use today. In addition, new studies are emerging which indicate that the antidiabetic properties of all ARBs may not be the same.

A variety of clinical trials with ARBs have been reported in which the incidence of new-onset type 2 diabetes has been examined post hoc or as a secondary end point. In reviewing these studies, the trials that have compared ARBs to other antihypertensive drugs (Table 6.1) should be distinguished from those that have compared ARBs to placebos (Table 6.2). Such a distinction is required to assess whether ARBs merely have less potential to promote diabetes than other antihypertensive drugs or actually have the potential to protect against diabetes.

In all of the relevant studies in which ARBs have been compared to other antihypertensive drugs, the incidence of new-onset type 2 diabetes has been significantly lower in the patients treated with ARBs (see Table 6.1). In the LIFE trial, the incidence of new-onset type 2 diabetes was significantly lower in hypertensive subjects treated with losartan than in those treated with atenolol.[4] In the VALUE trial, the incidence of new-onset type 2 diabetes was significantly lower in hypertensive subjects treated with valsartan than in those treated with amlodipine.[6] In the ALPINE trial, the incidence of new-onset type 2 diabetes was significantly lower in the

Table 6.1
Clinical trials comparing antidiabetic effects of ARBs to other antihypertensive drugs (without placebo controls).

Trial	Treatment	Follow-up	Incidence of new diabetes	p value
LIFE	Losartan vs atenolol	4.8 years	6% vs 8% (241/4006 vs 319/3992)	<0.001
VALUE	Valsartan vs amlodipine	4.2 years	13.1% vs 16.4% (690/5267 vs 845/5152)	<0.0001
ALPINE	Candesartan ± felodipine vs hydrochlorothiazide ± atenolol	1 year	0.5% vs 4.3% (1/195 vs 8/188)	0.03

Table 6.2
Clinical trials comparing antidiabetic effects of ARBs to placebo.

Trial	Treatment	Follow-up	Incidence of new diabetes	p value
CHARM Preserved	Candesartan vs placebo	~3 years	4.4% vs 7.1% (47/1080 vs 77/1086)	0.005
CHARM Alternative	Candesartan vs placebo	~3 years	6% vs 7.1% (44/735 vs 53/745)	ns
CHARM Added	Candesartan vs placebo	~3.5 years	8% vs 8.1% (72/900 vs 72/890)	ns
SCOPE Added	Candesartan vs placebo	~3.7 years	4.3% vs 5.3% (93/2168 vs 115/2175)	ns

hypertensive patients randomized to candesartan (alone or in combination with felodipine) than in those randomized to hydrochlorothiazide (alone or in combination with atenolol).[11] Although the 1-year ALPINE study involved only 392 patients and relatively few cases of new-onset diabetes were observed during the course of the trial, both the LIFE and VALUE studies followed thousands of patients for at least 4 years and hundreds of cases of new-onset diabetes developed during each trial. In these large trials, the incidence of new-onset diabetes was approximately 20–25% lower in the subjects randomized to ARBs than in those randomized to the other antihypertensive drugs.

Given the consistent results of the LIFE, VALUE, and ALPINE trials and given that these studies involved different ARBs and different antihypertensive agents, it appears quite possible that the incidence of new-onset diabetes is lower in hypertensive subjects treated with ARBs as a class than in those treated with other antihypertensive drugs. Nevertheless, these trials leave open a number of major questions:

1. Is the lower incidence of new-onset diabetes in the patients treated with ARBs related to an antidiabetic effect of angiotensin II receptor blockade or to a prodiabetic effect of the comparator agents, or both?
2. Will the lower rate of new-onset diabetes in patients treated with ARBs be sustained over longer periods of time?
3. Is the rate of new-onset diabetes the same regardless of which ARB is used?
4. Will the lower rate of new-onset diabetes in patients treated with ARBs vs other antihypertensive drugs translate into lower rates of morbidity or mortality or into better quality of life?

The answers to these questions will require long-term, randomized, placebo-controlled trials using a variety of ARBs. In the absence of such data, however, some insight into these questions may be gained from the limited clinical data available from studies involving either placebo controls or head-to-head comparisons of the metabolic effects of different ARBs.

In contrast to the LIFE, VALUE, and ALPINE trials, the CHARM and SCOPE trials included placebo controls and investigated whether angiotensin receptor blockade could actually reduce the risk for new-onset diabetes as a secondary end point (see Table 6.2).[5,12–14] In the CHARM Preserved trial, the incidence of new-onset type 2 diabetes was significantly lower in subjects given candesartan than in those given placebo.[5] However, in the other placebo-controlled trials, including CHARM Alternative, CHARM Added, and SCOPE Added, there was no significant difference in the incidence of new-onset diabetes in subjects given candesartan compared with controls (see Table 6.2).[12–14] Nevertheless, when the results of all three CHARM studies were combined, the rate of new-onset diabetes was lower in the candesartan-treated patients than in patients given placebo.[15]

While the results of the placebo-controlled trials are intriguing, they have been less consistent than those in which ARBs have been compared with other antihypertensive drugs. Moreover, because all of the placebo-controlled trials reported so far have been performed with candesartan, they shed no light on whether different ARBs might have different capacities to prevent diabetes. However, the results of two large-scale placebo-controlled trials that are currently being conducted with valsartan and telmisartan should provide useful information on the true antidiabetic properties of at least some additional ARBs. The NAVIGATOR trial is investigating whether the oral antidiabetic agent nateglinide or the ARB valsartan can prevent diabetes as a primary end point in individuals with impaired glucose tolerance who are at high risk for cardiovascular events.[16] This randomized, double-blind, placebo-controlled trial involves over 7000 subjects, and the diabetes end point will be assessed 3 years after the last trial participant is enrolled. In the ONTARGET trial, subjects at increased risk for cardiovascular events, including many subjects at increased risk for diabetes, have been randomized to receive either telmisartan, ramipril, or a combination of telmisartan and ramipril.[17,18] In the companion TRANSCEND trial, subjects that are intolerant of ACE inhibitors but are otherwise similar to those enrolled in ONTARGET have been randomized to placebo or telmisartan. Reduction in the incidence of new-onset type 2 diabetes will be a secondary end point in both the ONTARGET and TRANSCEND trials.[17,18]

While awaiting the results of clinical trials prospectively designed to test whether ARBs can actually prevent diabetes, it may be instructive to examine the results of studies investigating the effects of ARBs on glucose and lipid metabolism. For example, in the CROSS study and in the ALPINE study, measurements of serum insulin, glucose, and lipid levels were obtained before and after the administration of either candesartan or hydrochlorothiazide.[11,19] Hypertensive subjects in the CROSS trial were studied before and after 12 weeks of therapy, whereas hypertensive subjects in the ALPINE trial were studied before and after 1 year of therapy. Candesartan had little or no effect on serum insulin, glucose, triglyceride, or cholesterol levels in either the CROSS trial or the ALPINE trial. However, increases in glucose, insulin, and triglyceride levels, and decreases in HDL cholesterol levels were observed in hydrochlorothiazide-treated patients in the ALPINE study.[11] Little or no changes in glucose, insulin, or lipid levels were observed in hydrochlorothiazide-treated patients in the CROSS study, perhaps owing to the short-term nature of the trial.[19] Both the short-term CROSS study and the longer-term ALPINE study indicate that candesartan has little or no effect on glucose or lipid levels in patients with hypertension. Although candesartan treatment appeared to improve an indirect estimate of insulin action in the CROSS study, it failed to show any effect on the HOMA index of insulin resistance in the longer-term ALPINE study. Thus, to the extent that candesartan may have contributed to increases in insulin sensitivity in the short-term CROSS study, the increases in insulin sensitivity did not translate into any improvements in serum glucose or lipid levels and it is unclear how long any such effects on insulin sensitivity might be sustained. At most, one might conclude from the CROSS and ALPINE studies that in patients with hypertension, candesartan therapy is 'metabolically neutral.'

Clinical studies with a variety of ARBs have yielded inconsistent results on glucose and lipid metabolism, thereby underscoring the question: do some ARBs have greater metabolic benefits than others and if so, why (Table 6.3)? For example, Derosa et al recently compared the metabolic effects of telmisartan, 40 mg/day, to eprosartan 600 mg/day, in 119 patients with mild hypertension and type 2 diabetes.[20] After 12 months of once-daily treatment, this low dose of telmisartan produced a significant 25–30% reduction in triglyceride concentrations compared with baseline; in contrast, neither eprosartan nor placebo had any detectable effect on triglyceride levels. Neither agent appeared to affect glucose levels in this study. In patients with type 2 diabetes and hypertension, Honjo et al found that administration of telmisartan, 40 mg/day for 3 months, was associated with modest reductions in hemoglobin A_{1c} levels, whereas candesartan, 8 mg/day, was not.[21] Miura et al reported that in patients with type 2 diabetes and hypertension, switching from either candesartan 8 mg/day or valsartan 80 mg/day, to 40 mg/day of telmisartan, was associated with significant improvements in fasting insulin, triglycerides, adiponectin, and high-sensitivity C-reactive protein levels.[22] Vitale et al found that in a 3-month randomized, parallel-group trial comparing telmisartan 80 mg/day with losartan 50 mg/day in 40 patients with metabolic syndrome, telmisartan produced significant reductions from baseline in fasting glucose, hemoglobin A_{1c} levels, insulin resistance, and insulin levels, whereas losartan did not.[23] Insulin clamp studies in hypertensive patients treated with 50 mg/day of losartan for 4–6 weeks have yielded inconsistent results, with some showing improvements in insulin sensitivity and others showing little or no effect on insulin sensitivity.[24-30]

Taken together, the results of head-to-head comparisons of different ARBs suggest that the metabolic effects of all ARBs may not be the same and that certain ARBs such as telmisartan may have potential for causing greater metabolic benefits than others (see Table 6.3). One possible explanation for this is that the metabolic effects of different ARBs are dose-dependent and that higher doses of losartan, candesartan, or valsartan might be required to achieve the

Table 6.3
Clinical studies designed to compare the metabolic effects of different ARBs.

Treatment	Reference	Duration	Patients	Metabolic changes
Telmisartan 40mg/day vs eprosartan 600mg/day	20	12 months	HTN & type 2 DM	Telmisartan improved triglycerides
Telmisartan 40mg/day vs candesartan 8mg/day	21	3 months	HTN & type 2 DM	Telmisartan improved hemoglobin A_{1c}
Telmisartan 40mg/day vs candesartan 8mg/day or valsartan 80mg/day	22	3 months	HTN & type 2 DM	Telmisartan improved insulin, triglycerides, adiponectin, and hs-CRP
Telmisartan 80mg/day vs losartan 50mg/day	23	3 months	Metabolic syndrome	Telmisartan improved fasting glucose, insulin, and hemoglobin A1c

HTN, hypertension; DM, diabetes mellitus; hs-CRP, high-sensitivity C-reactive protein.

same degree of metabolic improvement as seen with telmisartan. In most of the clinical studies conducted to date, the ARB doses have been on the low side, and it is possible that beneficial metabolic effects of some ARBs might be observed at higher doses. For example, in contrast to the negative results of Vitale et al performed with 50 mg/day losartan, other investigators have reported metabolic benefits with 100 mg/day of losartan. In a placebo-controlled study in patients with hypertension and hypercholesterolemia, Koh et al reported that 100 mg/day of losartan was associated with a significant increase in adiponectin levels and a significant decrease in insulin levels without any change in glucose levels.[31] However, in addition to dosing issues, it is also possible that some ARBs may have greater metabolic benefits than others, owing to different effects on the mechanisms that mediate the antidiabetic effects of these drugs.

Mechanisms

The mechanisms that may mediate the antidiabetic effects of ARBs can be divided into two categories: those that depend on blockade of the adverse metabolic effects of angiotensin II (Table 6.4) and those that do not (Table 6.5). Many in-vitro experiments and studies in animals and in humans have indicated a possible relationship between adverse metabolic effects of angiotensin II and the pathogenesis of insulin resistance. For example, excess angiotensin II may promote impaired glucose metabolism through its effects on insulin signaling pathways, tissue blood flow, oxidative stress, potassium balance, sympathetic activity, pancreatic function, and adipogenesis.[25,32–47] Thus, blockade of these adverse metabolic effects of angiotensin II via blockade of the angiotensin II type 1 receptor might well be expected to lead to improvements in glucose and lipid metabolism. Indeed, to the extent that angiotensin II-dependent mechanisms promote insulin resistance, one might expect all drugs that effectively interfere with

Table 6.4
Antidiabetic mechanisms of ARBs related to blocking adverse effects of angiotensin II.

Improved insulin signaling
Increased tissue blood flow
Decreased oxidative stress
Decreased sympathetic activity
Increased potassium levels
Improved pancreatic function
Increased adipogenesis

Table 6.5
Antidiabetic mechanisms of ARBs that are not related to blocking adverse effects of angiotensin II.

Increased activity of bradykinin/nitric oxide pathways
Activation of PPAR-γ *

*Not a property of all ARBs.

either the generation or action of angiotensin II to be relatively useful in improving insulin sensitivity and preventing type 2 diabetes. The fact that both ARBs and ACE inhibitors show promise for preventing diabetes is consistent with the notion that interference with the adverse metabolic effects of angiotensin II is an important determinant of the antidiabetic effects of these drugs. However, further studies will be required to delineate the relative importance of angiotensin II receptor blockade per se versus other mechanisms that may mediate the antidiabetic effects of different ARBs.

Recent studies have suggested that some ARBs may have antidiabetic properties that involve more than just blockade of the adverse metabolic effects of angiotensin II.[48–50] The two main antidiabetic mechanisms that do not involve blocking adverse metabolic actions of angiotensin II are the effects on bradykinin/nitric oxide pathways and the effects on the peroxisome proliferator-activated receptor gamma (PPAR-γ) (see Table 6.5). Bradykinin/nitric oxide pathways have previously been implicated in the antidiabetic effects of ACE inhibitors as these agents interfere with bradykinin degradation and increase bradykinin levels.[46,51–59] Increases in bradykinin can increase nitric oxide activity, which in turn can promote increases in insulin sensitivity through effects on the GLUT4 glucose transporter.[59] ARBs may also have effects on bradykinin/nitric oxide pathways that could lead to increases in GLUT4 activity. Blockade of angiotensin II type 1 (AT$_1$) receptors by AT$_1$ receptor antagonists leads to feedback increases in circulating levels of angiotensin II that in turn may stimulate angiotensin II type 2 (AT$_2$) receptors.[60] AT$_2$ receptor activation may increase nitric oxide either directly, or indirectly via stimulation of bradykinin levels and the B$_2$ receptor.[60,61] Although bradykinin/nitric oxide pathways have been strongly implicated in the metabolic effects of ACE inhibitors, the extent to which bradykinin/nitric oxide pathways contribute to improved insulin sensitivity with ARBs remains to be determined.

Assuming that both enhancement of bradykinin/nitric oxide activity and interference with the adverse metabolic effects of angiotensin II contribute to the antidiabetic effects of ARBs, how does one explain the apparent variation in the ability of different ARBs to affect glucose and lipid metabolism? Notwithstanding the relatively similar capacity of different ARBs to lower blood pressure, it is possible that different ARBs vary in their ability to affect angiotensin II or bradykinin/nitric oxide-mediated changes in glucose and lipid metabolism. It is also possible that ARBs differ in their effects on antidiabetic mechanisms that are unrelated to effects on the renin–angiotensin system or bradykinin/nitric oxide pathways.

The tacit assumption that underlies the interpretation of most studies involving ARBs is that these molecules interact only with the angiotensin II receptor and, therefore, most if not all of their biologic properties are secondary to angiotensin II receptor blockade. However, this assumption appears to be incorrect because some ARBs have recently been found to activate PPAR-γ, a nuclear hormone receptor that is known to play a critical role in both carbohydrate and lipid metabolism.[48–50]

In cellular PPAR-γ transactivation assays, the ARB telmisartan has been found to produce significant activation of PPAR-γ when tested at concentrations that may be achieved in plasma following administration of doses used for the treatment of essential hypertension.[48] By contrast, the other commercially available ARBs – losartan and its main metabolite EXP3174, eprosartan, candesartan, valsartan, olmesartan, and irbesartan – appear to have little ability to activate PPAR-γ when tested at the same concentrations, although higher concentrations of irbesartan and losartan are able to cause some activation of the receptor.[48,50] High concentrations of a minor losartan metabolite, EXP3179, have also been reported to activate PPAR-γ in vitro, but the relevance of this observation to the in-vivo situation is unclear.[62] In contrast to the other commercially available ARBs, telmisartan is a more potent, selective PPAR-γ agonist, activating the receptor to 25–30% of the maximum level achieved by conventional full agonists such as pioglitazone and rosiglitazone. The concentration of telmisartan that yielded its half-maximal activation of the PPAR-γ receptor (EC_{50}) was approximately 4.5 μM, which is of a similar order of magnitude to that of pioglitazone ($EC_{50} = 1.5$ μM). Furthermore, the effect was specific for PPAR-γ, with telmisartan exhibiting no activation of PPAR-α or PPAR-δ when tested at concentrations achieved in plasma with usual oral dosing for hypertension. Given the well-known antidiabetic effects of thiazolidinedione ligands of PPAR-γ, these findings raise the distinct possibility that some ARBs such as telmisartan may be exerting antidiabetic effects through activation of PPAR-γ.

Clinical significance

It is well established that a diagnosis of diabetes puts many burdens on the patient and that diabetes increases morbidity and mortality. Thus, it would seem intuitively obvious that antihypertensive agents that are associated with a decreased risk for diabetes would be more desirable than otherwise equally effective antihypertensive drugs that do not protect against diabetes or actually increase the risk for diabetes. Nevertheless, considerable controversy exists regarding the clinical significance of differences in the incidence of diabetes among patients treated with different antihypertensive agents.[63–67]

Although trial results regarding the clinical significance of the antidiabetic effects of ARBs are limited, it may be instructive to consider data relating to other antihypertensive drugs. In the ALLHAT trial, a greater rate of new-onset diabetes in patients treated with chlorthalidone vs amlodipine or lisinopril 'did not translate into more cardiovascular events or into higher all cause mortality in the chlorthalidone group' during an average follow-up of 4.9 years.[3] However, it is possible that the lower systolic blood pressures achieved in the chlorthalidone group might have counterveiled the increased cardiovascular risk otherwise conferred by the new-onset diabetes. In the PIUMA study, which corrected for multiple risk factors including blood pressure, the relative risk for cardiovascular events was significantly increased in patients who developed diabetes during antihypertensive therapy vs those persistently free of diabetes.[65]

The notion that new-onset diabetes during hypertension therapy does not influence cardiovascular morbidity or mortality has also been criticized, owing to lack of relevant studies of sufficiently long duration.[64] For example, in the VALUE study with a follow-up period of 4 years, the lower rate of new-onset diabetes in the valsartan-treated patients vs the amlodipine-treated patients did not translate into improved cardiovascular outcomes.[6] However, it has been proposed that 10–15 years may be required before the increased risk of new-onset diabetes becomes apparent and that studies of very long duration will be required to show benefits from the antidiabetic effects of certain antihypertensive drugs.

Recently, cardiovascular outcomes after a mean follow-up of 14.3 years were reported from the SHEP trial in which the rate of new-onset diabetes was significantly greater in patients randomized to chlorthalidone than in those randomized to placebo.[66] The rates of all-cause mortality and cardiovascular mortality were significantly greater in placebo-treated subjects who developed new-onset diabetes than in placebo-treated subjects who did not develop diabetes. In contrast, the rates of all-cause mortality and cardiovascular mortality were not significantly different between chlorthalidone-treated subjects who developed new-onset diabetes and chlorthalidone-treated subjects who did not develop diabetes. Thus, new-onset diabetes was not associated with increased mortality when the patients were receiving chlorthalidone.

However, other potential problems associated with a diagnosis of diabetes were not examined. In addition, chlorthalidone was associated with reduced cardiovascular mortality rates in patients who had diabetes at baseline but not in patients who developed diabetes during the course of therapy. Thus, an alternative way of interpreting the SHEP trial results is that chlorthalidone confers protection against cardiovascular mortality in patients with pre-existing diabetes but not in those who develop new-onset diabetes during therapy. However, it is also possible that this post hoc analysis of the SHEP trial was underpowered to detect all the relationships between new-onset diabetes, chlorthalidone, and cardiovascular mortality. Failure to detect adverse effects of new-onset diabetes in patients given chlorthalidone or to detect protective effects of chlorthalidone vs placebo in patients with new-onset diabetes may have been due to sample size limitations. Finally, the results of the SHEP trial do not indicate whether long-term cardiovascular outcomes will be different in hypertensive subjects who are treated with a diuretic or β-blocker and develop diabetes during therapy vs hypertensive subjects who are treated with an ARB and do not develop diabetes.

Even if lower rates of new-onset diabetes in ARB-treated patients fail to translate into reduced mortality rates in long-term clinical trials, one must still consider the quality of life issues and potential benefits of reducing a host of other problems that often attend the diagnosis of diabetes. Although the clinical significance of the antidiabetic effects of any of the ARBs remains to be determined, some benefits may be anticipated even if the metabolic effects do not translate directly into reduced rates of cardiovascular mortality or all-cause mortality.

References

1. Gress TW, Nieto FJ, Shahar E, Wofford MR, Brancati FL. Hypertension and antihypertensive therapy as risk factors for type 2 diabetes mellitus. Atherosclerosis Risk in Communities Study. N Engl J Med 2000; 342(13):905–12.
2. Hansson L, Lindholm LH, Niskanen L et al. Effect of angiotensin-converting-enzyme inhibition compared with conventional therapy on cardiovascular morbidity and mortality in hypertension: the Captopril Prevention Project (CAPPP) randomised trial. Lancet 1999; 353(9153):611–16.
3. Major outcomes in high-risk hypertensive patients randomized to angiotensin-converting enzyme inhibitor or calcium channel blocker vs diuretic: The Antihypertensive and Lipid-Lowering Treatment to Prevent Heart Attack Trial (ALLHAT). JAMA 2002; 288(23):2981–97.
4. Lindholm LH, Ibsen H, Borch-Johnsen K et al. Risk of new-onset diabetes in the Losartan Intervention For Endpoint reduction in hypertension study. J Hypertens 2002; 20(9):1879–86.
5. Yusuf S, Pfeffer MA, Swedberg K et al. Effects of candesartan in patients with chronic heart failure and preserved left-ventricular ejection fraction: the CHARM-Preserved Trial. Lancet 2003; 362(9386):777–81.
6. Julius S, Kjeldsen SE, Weber M et al. Outcomes in hypertensive patients at high cardiovascular risk treated with regimens based on valsartan or amlodipine: the VALUE randomized trial. Lancet 2004; 363:2022–31.
7. Opie LH, Schall R. Old antihypertensives and new diabetes. J Hypertens 2004; 22(8):1453–8.
8. Isomaa B, Almgren P, Tuomi T et al. Cardiovascular morbidity and mortality associated with the metabolic syndrome. Diabetes Care 2001; 24(4):683–9.
9. Lakka HM, Laaksonen DE, Lakka TA et al. The metabolic syndrome and total and cardiovascular disease mortality in middle-aged men. JAMA 2002; 288(21):2709–16.
10. Laaksonen DE, Lakka HM, Niskanen LK et al. Metabolic syndrome and development of diabetes mellitus: application and validation of recently suggested definitions of the metabolic syndrome in a prospective cohort study. Am J Epidemiol 2002; 156(11):1070–7.
11. Lindholm LH, Persson M, Alaupovic P et al. Metabolic outcome during 1 year in newly detected hypertensives: results of the Antihypertensive Treatment and Lipid Profile in a North of Sweden Efficacy Evaluation (ALPINE study). J Hypertens 2003; 21(8):1563–74.
12. Granger CB, McMurray JJ, Yusuf S et al. Effects of candesartan in patients with chronic heart failure and reduced left-ventricular systolic function intolerant to angiotensin-converting-enzyme inhibitors: the CHARM-Alternative trial. Lancet 2003; 362(9386):772–6.
13. McMurray JJ, Ostergren J, Swedberg K et al. Effects of candesartan in patients with chronic heart failure and reduced left-ventricular systolic function taking angiotensin-converting-enzyme inhibitors: the CHARM-Added trial. Lancet 2003; 362(9386):767–71.
14. Lithell H, Hansson L, Skoog I et al. The Study on Cognition and Prognosis in the Elderly (SCOPE): principal results of a randomized double-blind intervention trial. J Hypertens 2003; 21(5):875–86.
15. Pfeffer MA, Swedberg K, Granger CB et al. Effects of candesartan on mortality and morbidity in patients with chronic heart failure: the CHARM-Overall programme. Lancet 2003; 362(9386):759–66.
16. Prisant LM. Preventing type II diabetes mellitus. J Clin Pharmacol 2004; 44(4):406–13.
17. Zimmermann M, Unger T. Challenges in improving prognosis and therapy: the Ongoing Telmisartan Alone and in Combination with Ramipril Global End point Trial Programme. Expert Opin Pharmacother 2004; 5(5):1201–8.
18. Teo K, Yusuf S, Sleight P et al. Rationale, design, and baseline characteristics of 2 large, simple randomized trials evaluating telmisartan, ramipril, and their combination in high-risk patients: the Ongoing Telmisartan Alone and in Combination with Ramipril Global Endpoint Trial/Telmisartan

Randomized Assessment Study in ACE Intolerant Subjects with Cardiovascular Disease (ONTARGET/TRANSCEND) trials. Am Heart J 2004; 148:52–61.

19. Grassi G, Seravalle G, Dell'Oro R et al. Comparative effects of candesartan and hydrochlorothiazide on blood pressure, insulin sensitivity, and sympathetic drive in obese hypertensive individuals: results of the CROSS study. J Hypertens 2003; 21(9):1761–9.

20. Derosa G, Ragonesi PD, Mugellini A, Ciccarelli L, Fogari R. Effects of telmisartan compared with eprosartan on blood pressure control, glucose metabolism and lipid profile in hypertensive, type 2 diabetic patients: a randomized, double-blind, placebo-controlled 12-month study. Hypertens Res 2004; 27(7):457–64.

21. Honjo S, Nichi Y, Wada Y, Hamamoto Y, Koshiyama H. Possible beneficial effect of telmisartan on glycemic control in diabetic subjects. Diabetes Care 2005; 28(2):498.

22. Miura Y, Yamamoto N, Tsunekawa S et al. Replacement of valsartan and candesartan by telmisartan in hypertensive patients with type 2 diabetes: metabolic and antiatherogenic consequences. Diabetes Care 2005; 28(3):757–8.

23. Vitale C, Mercuro G, Castiglioni C et al. Metabolic effect of telmisartan and losartan in hypertensive patients with metabolic syndrome. Cardiovasc Diabetol 2005; 4:6.

24. Laakso M, Karjalainen L, Lempiainen-Kuosa P. Effects of losartan on insulin sensitivity in hypertensive subjects. Hypertension 1996; 28(3):392–6.

25. Paolisso G, Tagliamonte MR, Gambardella A et al. Losartan mediated improvement in insulin action is mainly due to an increase in non-oxidative glucose metabolism and blood flow in insulin-resistant hypertensive patients. J Hum Hypertens 1997; 11(5):307–12.

26. Fogari R, Zoppi A, Corradi L et al. Comparative effects of lisinopril and losartan on insulin sensitivity in the treatment of non diabetic hypertensive patients. Br J Clin Pharmacol 1998; 46(5):467–71.

27. Fogari R, Zoppi A, Preti P et al. Differential effects of ACE-inhibition and angiotensin II antagonism on fibrinolysis and insulin sensitivity in hypertensive postmenopausal women. Am J Hypertens 2001; 14(9 Pt 1):921–6.

28. Fogari R, Zoppi A, Lazzari P et al. ACE inhibition but not angiotensin II antagonism reduces plasma fibrinogen and insulin resistance in overweight hypertensive patients. J Cardiovasc Pharmacol 1998; 32(4):616–20.

29. Moan A, Hoieggen A, Seljeflot I et al. The effect of angiotensin II receptor antagonism with losartan on glucose metabolism and insulin sensitivity. J Hypertens 1996; 14(9):1093–7.

30. Moan A, Risanger T, Eide I, Kjeldsen SE. The effect of angiotensin II receptor blockade on insulin sensitivity and sympathetic nervous system activity in primary hypertension. Blood Press 1994; 3(3):185–8.

31. Koh KK, Quon MJ, Han SH et al. Additive beneficial effects of losartan combined with simvastatin in the treatment of hypercholesterolemic, hypertensive patients. Circulation 2004; 110(24):3687–92.

32. Ogihara T, Asano T, Ando K et al. Angiotensin II-induced insulin resistance is associated with enhanced insulin signaling. Hypertension 2002; 40(6):872–9.

33. Velloso LA, Folli F, Sun XJ et al. Cross-talk between the insulin and angiotensin signaling systems. Proc Natl Acad Sci USA 1996; 93(22):12490–5.

34. Folli F, Saad MJ, Velloso L et al. Crosstalk between insulin and angiotensin II signalling systems. Exp Clin Endocrinol Diabetes 1999; 107(2):133–9.

35. Folli F, Kahn CR, Hansen H, Bouchie JL, Feener EP. Angiotensin II inhibits insulin signaling in aortic smooth muscle cells at multiple levels. A potential role for serine phosphorylation in insulin/angiotensin II crosstalk. J Clin Invest 1997; 100(9):2158–69.

36. Nawano M, Anai M, Funaki M et al. Imidapril, an angiotensin-converting enzyme inhibitor, improves insulin sensitivity by enhancing signal transduction via insulin receptor substrate proteins and improving vascular resistance in the Zucker fatty rat. Metabolism 1999; 48(10):1248–55.

37. Andreozzi F, Laratta E, Sciacqua A, Perticone F, Sesti G. Angiotensin II impairs the insulin signaling pathway promoting production of nitric oxide by inducing phosphorylation of insulin receptor substrate-1 on Ser312 and Ser616 in human umbilical vein endothelial cells. Circ Res 2004; 94(9):1211–18.

38. Scheen AJ. Prevention of type 2 diabetes mellitus through inhibition of the renin–angiotensin system. Drugs 2004; 64(22):2537–65.

39. Krutzfeldt J, Raasch W, Klein HH. Ramipril increases the protein level of skeletal muscle IRS-1 and alters protein tyrosine phosphatase activity in spontaneously hypertensive rats. Naunyn Schmiedebergs Arch Pharmacol 2000; 362(1):1–6.

40. Shiuchi T, Iwai M, Li HS et al. Angiotensin II type-1 receptor blocker valsartan enhances insulin sensitivity in skeletal muscles of diabetic mice. Hypertension 2004; 43(5):1003–10.

41. Tikellis C, Wookey PJ, Candido R et al. Improved islet morphology after blockade of the renin–angiotensin system in the ZDF rat. Diabetes 2004; 53(4):989–97.

42. Janke J, Engeli S, Gorzelniak K, Luft FC, Sharma AM. Mature adipocytes inhibit in vitro differentiation of human preadipocytes via angiotensin type 1 receptors. Diabetes 2002; 51(6):1699–707.

43. Sharma AM, Janke J, Gorzelniak K, Engeli S, Luft FC. Angiotensin blockade prevents type 2 diabetes by formation of fat cells. Hypertension 2002; 40(5):609–11.

44. Fliser D, Dikow R, Demukaj S, Ritz E. Opposing effects of angiotensin II on muscle and renal blood flow under euglycemic conditions. J Am Soc Nephrol 2000; 11(11):2001–6.

45. Carlsson PO, Berne C, Jansson L. Angiotensin II and the endocrine pancreas: effects on islet blood flow and insulin secretion in rats. Diabetologia 1998; 41(2):127–33.

46. Bernobich E, de Angelis L, Lerin C, Bellini G. The role of the angiotensin system in cardiac glucose homeostasis: therapeutic implications. Drugs 2002; 62(9):1295–314.

47. McFarlane SI, Kumar A, Sowers JR. Mechanisms by which angiotensin-converting enzyme inhibitors prevent diabetes and cardiovascular disease. Am J Cardiol 2003; 91(12A):30H–7H.

48. Benson SC, Pershadsingh HA, Ho CI et al. Identification of telmisartan as a unique angiotensin II receptor antagonist with selective PPARgamma-modulating activity. Hypertension 2004; 43:993–1002.

49. Kurtz TW, Pravenec M. Antidiabetic mechanisms of angiotensin-converting enzyme inhibitors and angiotensin II receptor antagonists: beyond the renin–angiotensin system. J Hypertens 2004; 22(12):2253–61.

50. Schupp M, Janke J, Clasen R, Unger T, Kintscher U. Angiotensin type 1 receptor blockers induce peroxisome proliferator-activated receptor-gamma activity. Circulation 2004; 109(17):2054–7.

51. Tomiyama H, Kushiro T, Abeta H et al. Kinins contribute to the improvement of insulin sensitivity during treatment with angiotensin converting enzyme inhibitor. Hypertension 1994; 23(4):450–5.

52. Rosenthal T, Erlich Y, Rosenmann E, Cohen A. Effects of enalapril, losartan, and verapamil on blood pressure and glucose metabolism in the Cohen–Rosenthal diabetic hypertensive rat. Hypertension 1997; 29(6):1260–4.

53. Henriksen EJ, Jacob S. Effects of captopril on glucose transport activity in skeletal muscle of obese Zucker rats. Metabolism 1995; 44(2):267–72.

54. Shiuchi T, Cui TX, Wu L et al. ACE inhibitor improves insulin resistance in diabetic mouse via bradykinin and NO. Hypertension 2002; 40(3):329–34.

55. Damas J, Hallet C, Lefebvre PJ. Changes in blood glucose and plasma insulin levels induced by bradykinin in anaesthetized rats. Br J Pharmacol 2001; 134(6):1312–18.

56. Kudoh A, Matsuki A. Effects of angiotensin-converting enzyme inhibitors on glucose uptake. Hypertension 2000; 36(2):239–44.

57. Chow L, De Gasparo M, Levens N. Improved glucose metabolism following blockade of angiotensin converting enzyme but not angiotensin AT1 receptors. Eur J Pharmacol 1995; 282(1–3):77–86.

58. Duka I, Shenouda S, Johns C et al. Role of the B(2) receptor of bradykinin in insulin sensitivity. Hypertension 2001; 38(6):1355–60.

59. Young ME, Radda GK, Leighton B. Nitric oxide stimulates glucose transport and metabolism in rat skeletal muscle in vitro. Biochem J 1997; 322 (Pt 1):223–8.

60. Carey RM. Update on the role of the AT2 receptor. Curr Opin Nephrol Hypertens 2005; 14(1):67–71.

61. Abadir PM, Carey RM, Siragy HM. Angiotensin AT2 receptors directly stimulate renal nitric oxide in bradykinin B2-receptor-null mice. Hypertension 2003; 42(4):600–4.

62. Krempl T, Schwedhelm E, Hornung D et al. Identification of EXP 3179 as selective PPAR gamma receptor agonist. Z Kardiol 2005; 94(Suppl 1):V62.

63. Elliott WJ. Differential effects of antihypertensive drugs on new-onset diabetes? Curr Hypertens Rep 2005; 7(4):249–56.

64. Aksnes TA, Reims HM, Kjeldsen SE, Mancia G. Antihypertensive treatment and new-onset diabetes mellitus. Curr Hypertens Rep 2005; 7(4):298–303.

65. Verdecchia P, Reboldi G, Angeli F et al. Adverse prognostic significance of new diabetes in treated hypertensive subjects. Hypertension 2004; 43(5):963–9.

66. Kostis JB, Wilson AC, Freudenberger RS et al. Long-term effect of diuretic-based therapy on fatal outcomes in subjects with isolated systolic hypertension with and without diabetes. Am J Cardiol 2005; 95(1):29–35.

67. Messerli FH, Grossman E, Leonetti G. Antihypertensive therapy and new onset diabetes. J Hypertens 2004; 22(10):1845–7.

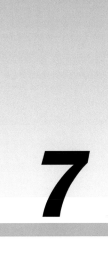

Angiotensin II antagonists, diabetes, and metabolic syndrome

Guido Grassi, Fosca Quarti Trevano, and Giuseppe Mancia

7

Introduction

Hypertension is a common comorbidity in diabetes mellitus and in the metabolic syndrome, potentiating the adverse effects of these abnormalities on cardiovascular structure, cardiovascular function and, by and large, on overall cardiovascular risk. This explains why in all the above-mentioned clinical conditions both US and European guidelines on antihypertensive treatment emphasize the importance of lowering blood pressure values well below usual goals, with the aim of achieving systolic/diastolic blood pressure values ≤130/80 mmHg.[1,2] Although all classes of antihypertensive drugs are effective in reducing high blood pressure values in diabetic or dysmetabolic patients, there is evidence that renin–angiotensin blockade by angiotensin II receptor antagonists, used alone or in combination with other drugs, may provide greater benefits than traditional agents by facilitating a more complete cardiovascular protection. This therapeutic approach allows us to:

- achieve a satisfactory blood pressure control in a large fraction of patients
- improve compliance to treatment by reducing or minimizing the side-effect profile of antihypertensive drugs and
- provide greater patient protection, particularly in patients displaying a high cardiovascular risk profile.

This chapter reviews the main objectives and features of the therapeutic approach to the clinical condition in which hypertension is complicated by diabetes, dyslipidemia, or metabolic syndrome. This is followed by a brief overview of the results obtained so far with the use of angiotensin II receptor blockers in the above-mentioned clinical conditions.

Blood pressure control in diabetic disease

Level A

Diabetes and hypertension frequently coexist, and their association provides additive increases in the risk of life-threatening cardiovascular events.[3] Quantification of this risk has been provided by different studies, that have documented a three- to fivefold increased incidence of fatal and non-fatal cardiovascular events in hypertensive patients displaying a type 2 diabetes mellitus.[4] The elevated cardiovascular risk of the diabetic hypertensive patients represents the background for tight blood pressure control in this clinical condition. Unequivocal evidence exists for a beneficial effect of blood pressure reduction on cardiovascular risk in type 2 diabetes. Evidence also exists indicating that these benefits can be achieved with all classes of antihypertensive drugs, including diuretics and β-blockers.[5,6] The benefits provided by angiotensin converting enzyme (ACE) inhibitors are well recognized and documented. Probably the strongest evidence for the cardiovascular benefits of this class of drugs in diabetic patients comes from the diabetic subgroup of the Heart Outcomes Prevention Evaluation (HOPE) trial,[7] in which the ACE inhibitor used, i.e. ramipril, facilitated a 37% reduction in the relative risk of cardiovascular fatal events, with a 24% decrease in the overall mortality rate. Finally, evidence exists in favor of the use of calcium channel blockers in diabetic hypertensives, although a perceived increase in the risk of coronary events might in some way limit a larger clinical use of these drugs in this clinical condition. This potential limitation, however, appears not to be supported by clinical trial results. In the Systolic Hypertension in Europe Trial (SHEP), for example, calcium antagonists treatment with nitrendipine caused a 70% reduction in cardiovascular mortality compared with placebo.[8] This result strengthens the concept that, regardless of the antihypertensive drug class employed, a reduction in blood pressure markedly decreases the incidence of cardiovascular events in diabetic hypertensives.

Level A

Several other features of antihypertensive treatment in diabetic disease deserve to be highlighted. First, as mentioned above, recent guidelines on antihypertensive treatment emphasize the need for an aggressive blood pressure reduction, with a therapeutic goal of systolic/diastolic values below 130/80 mmHg.[1,2] The reasons for this tight blood pressure reduction come from the evidence that

- diabetic patients, even when appropriately treated, display a cardiovascular risk higher than non-diabetics

- a continuous direct relationship exists between blood pressure values ranging from 113/70 to 169/100 mmHg and the incidence of myocardial infarction, and renal or cerebrovascular end points.[9]

It thus appears that lower blood pressure values are protective in diabetic hypertensives and that every effort should be taken to achieve these blood pressure goals in clinical practice. However, this appears to be a difficult task, even considering the results of the large-scale clinical trials published so far.[10] Indeed, in only half of these trials has the diastolic blood pressure been reduced to the target value of diabetics (<80 mmHg). The situation is even worse for systolic blood pressure, whose goal target (<130 mmHg) has not been achieved in any published study. Taken together, these findings support the notion that combination therapy is mandatory in hypertensive diabetics, which allows us to achieve blood pressure reduction of greater magnitude than that obtainable by using single drugs as monotherapy.

Level A

A second issue of clinical relevance is the differential effects of antihypertensive drug classes on cardiovascular outcome. Results of recently published studies support the notion that this is the case in diabetic hypertensives. The Irbesartan Diabetic Nephropathy Trial (IDNT),[11] for example, has shown that, although both irbesartan and amlodipine lower blood pressure to a similar extent, the angiotensin II receptor blocker only is capable of reducing the progression of the renal dysfunction to the end-stage renal disease. Further evidence of a differential effect of the various classes of antihypertensive drugs on cardiovascular outcome is provided by the results of the Losartan Intervention For Endpoint reduction in hypertension (LIFE) study,[12] which has shown, for similar blood pressure-lowering effects, a superiority of losartan vs atenolol in the reduction in cardiovascular deaths in a large group of hypertensive patients with or without diabetes. The evidence for a class effect on intermediate 'soft' end points is even stronger than for 'hard' end points. Angiotensin II receptor blockers have been shown to be more effective than other antihypertensive drugs in reducing proteinuria and other markers of renal damage in type 2 diabetes.[13] This finding, together with the evidence that ACE inhibitors and angiotensin II receptor blockers are particularly effective in preventing the progression of microalbuminuria to overt nephropathy in both type 1 and 2 diabetic patients, makes the drugs acting on the renin–angiotensin system not only the preferred compounds for initiating treatment but also the essential components of combination therapy.[13] The other drug(s) useful for the combination should be chosen among the other classes of antihypertensive compounds, taking into account

- the concomitant presence of target organ damage
- the need for obtaining greater cardiovascular protection and
- the anamnestic or instrumental evidence of previous coronary or cerebrovascular events.[2,13]

The choice should also be made taking into account the differential effects of antihypertensive drugs on new-onset diabetes,[7,14] as discussed in detail in the next section.

New-onset diabetes and angiotensin II antagonists

Level A

Although the hyperglycemic effects of β-blockers and diuretics in diabetes have been long known,[15] one of the most striking findings from recent clinical trials is the class-differential effects on new-onset diabetes (Figure 7.1). Calcium channel blockers, ACE inhibitors, and angiotensin II receptor blockers all have a remarkable impact on the risk of new-onset diabetes, which is less frequent when these drugs are administered compared with older drug classes over relatively short trial durations of 3–6 years. There has been some debate over whether such data reflect a prodiabetic effect of older drugs, or an antidiabetic effect of the new ones. Evidence from trials, however, also shows a reduced incidence of new-onset diabetes in patients treated with ACE inhibitors or angiotensin II receptor blockers as compared with placebo,[7,16,17] which suggests a 'true' antidiabetic effect of new drugs. In this regard, some other trials are important. This is the case in particular for the Valsartan Long-term Use Evaluation (VALUE) trial, which

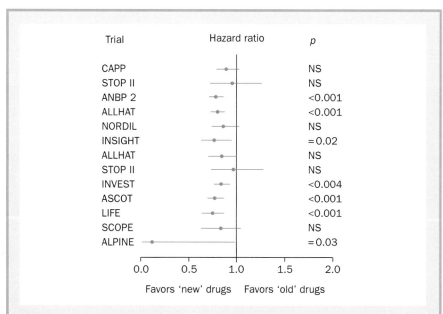

Figure 7.1

Comparison of 'new' and 'old' antihypertensive drugs for the outcome of new-onset diabetes mellitus in patients enrolled in different clinical trials. Data are expressed as hazard ratios. In the majority of the trials, new drugs appear to be less 'diabetogenic' than old ones.

showed a significant benefit for the angiotensin II receptor blocker valsartan over amlodipine, a metabolically neutral calcium channel blocker.[18]

Level B

A possibility which has been advanced is that the apparent diabetogenic effect of diuretics and β-blockers simply reflects a 'cosmetic' increase in blood glucose, with none of the adverse cardiovascular effects of true type 2 diabetes. Evidence that this is not the case has been provided by a study of 6886 hypertensive patients enrolled into a treatment program between 1973 and 1993 for an average of 6.3 years.[19] For most of the treatment period, diuretics or β-blockers were the first-line drugs. As expected, the incidence of cardiovascular disease during the study was significantly associated with raised blood glucose, whether measured at baseline or during treatment. Furthermore, patients who did not have raised blood glucose at baseline, but did have significantly raised levels (>7.75 mmol/L) at some point in the study, had a 50% increased incidence of cardiovascular disease, a rate very similar to that of patients with raised blood glucose at baseline. Furthermore, in another study, a treatment-induced increase in blood glucose in patients aged 50 years was the major predicting factor for the occurrence of myocardial infarction at the age of 60 years.[20] Based on these data, it seems that increases of blood glucose associated with antihypertensive treatment are just as serious as those that occur as a result of conventional risk factors.

Level A

There has been much speculation that blockade of the renin–angiotensin system can have a beneficial effect on the development of insulin resistance and the metabolic syndrome. Although the concept still remains controversial, data such as those of the VALUE trial[18] and from studies such as the Antihypertensive treatment and Lipid Profile In a North of Sweden Efficacy evaluation (ALPINE) study[21] are beginning to provide clinical support to the hypothesis. The ALPINE study compared candesartan cilexetil with hydrochlorothiazide in treatment-naive, non-diabetic hypertensives over a period of 1 year. Fasting serum glucose was unchanged by the angiotensin II receptor blocker (and increased by the diuretic) over the course of the study. As the metabolic syndrome is a paramount risk factor for diabetes, this strongly suggests that renin–angiotensin blockade provides a real protective effect on the risk of new diabetes.

Treatment of hypertension complicated by metabolic disease: role of angiotensin II antagonists

Level B

Dyslipidemia is frequent in hypertension, and is a major contributor to the occurrence of end-organ damage and cardiovascular events. In some conditions, such as in the initial forms of essential hypertension, the presence of hypercholesterolemia (i.e. the more common clinical expression of the dyslipidemic state as well as of the metabolic syndrome) may promote the progression of the disease itself, leading to stable hypertension. In these clinical conditions, an early and aggressive management of the hypercholesterolemic state has been shown not only to reduce cardiovascular complications but also to decrease the percentage of patients becoming affected with time by a stable form of hypertension.[22] A further variable complicating the clinical picture is represented by the evidence that the frequent association between hypercholesterolemia and hypertension is in both genders directly related to the severity of the hypertensive state, thus becoming more and more common as blood pressure increases over 160/100 mmHg.[23] This has been recently confirmed by the Pressioni Arteriose Monitorate E Loro Associazioni (PAMELA) study,[24] whose results have clearly documented that the close association between hypercholesterolemia and hypertension is manifest not only when clinic blood pressure values are considered but also when home or ambulatory blood pressure readings are taken into account (Figure 7.2). The results of the PAMELA study have also provided two

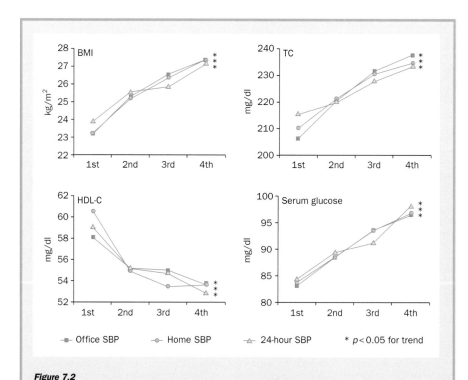

Figure 7.2

Relationship between body mass index (BMI), total cholesterol (TC), high-density lipoprotein cholesterol (HDL-C), serum glucose, and office, home, and 24-hour systolic blood pressure (SBP) values in the PAMELA Study. Data were analyzed taking into account quartiles (1st–4th) of blood pressure levels. Modified from Mancia et al.[24]

other pieces of information, by showing that cholesterol abnormalities (1) are closely associated to impaired fasting glucose, diabetes, overweight, or cigarette smoking and (2) are progressively more pronounced from the lowest to the highest quartiles of blood pressure values (see Figure 7.2).

Level B

European Guidelines on hypertension emphasize the importance of an aggressive treatment of both cardiovascular risk factors in the dyslipidemic hypertensive patient.[2] For primary prevention, current recommendations, based also on the results of the Heart Protection Study and Anglo-Scandinavian Outcome Trial-lipid Lowering Arm (ASCOT-LLA),[25,26] indicate reductions of total cholesterol below 190 mg/dl and low-density lipoprotein (LDL) cholesterol below 115 mg/dl as goals of the lipid-lowering treatment. In commenting on these targets of therapeutic intervention, two considerations should be made. First, in patients with established cardiovascular disease, diabetes, metabolic syndrome, or with an overall high cardiovascular risk profile, treatment goals for LDL cholesterol are lower.[27] Secondly, asymptomatic individuals at high cardiovascular risk may take benefit from further reduction of total cholesterol to values below 175 mg/dl and from further reduction of LDL cholesterol to below 100 mg/dl.[27] Blood pressure targets of antihypertensive treatment appear to be, in the dyslipidemic patient, almost superimposable to those recommended by guidelines for the hypertensive normolipidemic patient. Two important considerations should be made in this regard, however. The first one refers to the unique features of the cardiovascular risk profile of the metabolic syndrome. Indeed, a recent study of the PAMELA project has provided new insights on the prevalence as well as clinical significance of the metabolic syndrome, by showing that this condition:

- affects about 20% of the general population, its prevalence progressively increasing with age
- is associated with greater office, home, and ambulatory blood pressure levels, even when hypertensive patients are excluded and
- is frequently accompanied by target organ damage.

Level A

The second consideration refers to the blood pressure targets to be achieved when dyslipidemia and hypertension represent the components of the so-called metabolic syndrome, i.e. the clinical condition characterized by a high cardiovascular risk arising from a particular clustering of risk factors (Table 7.1).[28] Indeed, recent guidelines strongly recommend that in the presence of metabolic syndrome blood pressure values below 125/80 mmHg should be achieved.[28] These target blood pressure values appear, once again, difficult to achieve in clinical practice and require combination treatment strategies, possibly based on the association of drugs with antihypertensive as well as cardioprotective properties, such as calcium antagonists, ACE

Table 7.1

ATP III definition of metabolic syndrome based on the presence of three or more of the following components.

Central obesity	Waist circumference ≥102 cm in males and ≥88 cm in females
Impaired glucose metabolism	Fasting plasma glucose ≥110 mg/dl
Hypertriglyceridemia	≥150 mg/dl
Low LDL cholesterol	<40 mg/dl in males and <50 mg/dl in females
Blood pressure values	≥130/85 mmHg

inhibitors, or angiotensin II receptor blockers.[28] Specific data on the cardiovascular as well as on the metabolic effects of different antihypertensive drug classes in the hypertensive state complicating obesity as well as in the metabolic syndrome are lacking, however. This is the case also for angiotensin II receptor antagonists. A recent study performed by our group,[29] however, has provided some insights into the effects as well as the mechanisms of action of these drugs in obese hypertensive patients, a substantial proportion of whom are also affected by the metabolic syndrome. The study's goals were twofold:

- to obtain information on the effects of long-term treatment with the angiotensin II receptor blocker candesartan on the sympathetic and metabolic profile and
- to provide a comparative evaluation of the effects of angiotensin II antagonists vis-à-vis diuretic agents.

The main study results can be summarized as follows. First, in obese hypertensive patients with metabolic syndrome, angiotensin II receptor blockade exerts sustained sympathomoderating effects by reducing sympathetic nerve traffic (microneurographic recording) by about 30%. Secondly, these sympathoinhibitory properties were coupled with a clear-cut improvement in insulin sensitivity, as documented by the significant drug-induced reduction in the HOMA (Homeostatic Model Assessment) index values. Finally, opposite effects were seen with diuretic treatment (hydrochlorothiazide), which triggered a worsening in insulin sensitivity coupled with a slight increase in sympathetic cardiovascular drive (Figure 7.3).

Level B

Are the favorable metabolic effects of angiotensin II receptor antagonists class-specific? Although no data are available so far on this issue, it is likely that this is the case. This is because the results obtained with losartan or telmisartan administration in the LIFE and VALUE trials, respectively,[12,18] were similar to those observed in our study[29] as well as in the ALPINE study.[21] This does not mean, however, that some differences between drugs may exist. As discussed in detail in the previous chapter, it is likely that the agonistic activity toward the peroxisome proliferator-activated receptor-γ (PPAR-γ) displayed by some compounds such as telmisartan

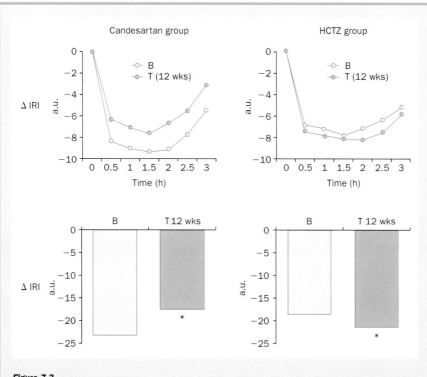

Figure 7.3

Changes in insulin resistance index (ΔIRI), expressed as overall points under the curves during the oral glucose load test (top panels) and as average values (bottom panels), induced by candesartan or hydrochlorothiazide (HCTZ) treatment. Data are shown before (B) and following 12 weeks of treatment (T) with either the angiotensin II antagonist or the diuretic drug. Asterisks (*) refer to the statistical significance between B and T. Modified from Grassi et al.[29] a.u., arbitrary unit.

may guarantee greater favorable metabolic effects, acting as insulin sensitizer.[30] Future studies, however, will be needed to clarify whether and to what extent the favorable metabolic effects of angiotensin II receptor antagonists result in a greater cardiovascular protection and a better cardiovascular outcome.

References

1. Chobanian AV, Bakris GL, Black HR et al. The Seventh Report of the Joint National Committee on Prevention, Detection, Evaluation and Treatment of High Blood Pressure: the JNC 7 Report. JAMA 2003; 289:2560–72.
2. Guidelines Committee 2003 European Society of Hypertension–European Society of Cardiology guidelines for the management of arterial hypertension. J Hypertens 2003; 21:1011–53.
3. Mancia G. The association of hypertension and diabetes: prevalence, cardiovascular risk and protection by blood pressure reduction. Acta Diabetol 2005; 42:517–25.
4. Stamler J, Vaccaro O, Neaton JD, Wentworth D. Diabetes, other risk factors and 12-yr cardiovascular

mortality for men screened in the Multiple Risk Factor Intervention Trial. Diabetes Care 1993; 16:434–44.

5. Curb JD, Pressel SL, Cutler JA et al. Effect of diuretic-based antihypertensive treatment on cardiovascular disease risk in older diabetic patients with isolated systolic hypertension. Systolic Hypertension in the Elderly Program Cooperative Research Group. JAMA 1996; 276:1886–92.

6. UK Prospective Diabetes Study Group. Efficacy of atenolol and captopril in reducing risk of macrovascular and microvascular complications in type 2 diabetes: UKPDS 39. BMJ 1998; 317:713–20.

7. Heart Outcomes Prevention Evaluation (HOPE) Study Investigators. Effects of ramipril on cardiovascular and microvascular outcomes in people with diabetes mellitus: results of the HOPE study and MICRO-HOPE substudy. Lancet 2000; 355:253–9.

8. Tuomilehto J, Rastenyte D, Birkenhager WH et al. Effects of calcium-channel blockade in older patients with diabetes and systolic hypertension: Systolic Hypertension in Europe Trial Investigators. N Engl J Med 1999; 340:677–84.

9. Zanchetti A, Hansson L, Menard J et al. Risk assessment and treatment benefit in intensively treated hypertensive patients of the Hypertension Optimal Treatment (HOT) study. J Hypertens 2001; 19:819–25.

10. Mancia G, Grassi G. Systolic and diastolic blood pressure control in antihypertensive drug trials. J Hypertens 2002; 20:1461–4.

11. Lewis EJ, Hunsicker LG, Clarke WR et al for the Collaborative Study Group. Renoprotective effect of the angiotensin-receptor antagonist irbesartan in patients with nephropathy due to type 2 diabetes. N Engl J Med 2001; 345:851–60.

12. Dahlof B, Devereux RB, Kjeldsen SE et al, for the LIFE Study Group. A paper by Lindholm LH et al. Cardiovascular morbidity and mortality in patients with diabetes in the Losartan Intervention For Endpoint reduction in hypertension study (LIFE): a randomised trial against atenolol. Lancet 2002; 359:1004–10.

13. American Diabetes Association Hypertension management in adults with diabetes. Diabetes Care 2004; 27(Suppl.1):65–7.

14. Mancia G, Zanchetti A, Grassi G. New onset diabetes and antihypertensive drugs. J Hypertens 2006; 24:3–10.

15. Struthers AD, Murphy MB, Dollery CT. Glucose tolerance during antihypertensive therapy in patients with diabetes mellitus. Hypertension 1985; 7:95–101.

16. Pfeffer MA, Swedberg K, Granger CB et al. Effects of candesartan on mortality and morbidity in patients with chronic heart failure: the CHARM – overall programme. Lancet 2003; 362:759–66.

17. Vermes E, Ducharme A, Bourassa MG et al. Enalapril reduces the incidence of diabetes in patients with chronic heart failure: insight from the Studies Of Left Ventricular Dysfunction (SOLVD). Circulation 2003; 107:1291–6.

18. Julius S, Kjeldsen SE, Weber M et al. Outcomes in hypertensive patients at high cardiovascular risk treated with regimens based on valsartan or amlodipine: the VALUE randomized trial. Lancet 2004; 363:2022–31.

19. Alderman MH, Cohen H, Madhavan S. Diabetes and cardiovascular events in hypertensive patients. Hypertension 1999; 33:1130–4.

20. Dunder K, Lind L, Zethelius B. Increase in blood glucose concentration during hypertensive treatment as a predictor of myocardial infarction: population based cohort study. BMJ 2003; 326:681–8.

21. Lindholm LH, Persson M, Alaupovic P et al. Metabolic outcome during 1 year in newly detected hypertensives: results of the Antihypertensive Treatment and Lipid Profile in a North of Sweden Efficacy Evaluation (ALPINE study). J Hypertens 2003; 21:1563–74.

22. Ekelund LG. Lowering lipids and the genesis of hypertension. Drugs 1988; 36(Suppl 3):21.

23. Muntner P, He J, Roccella EJ, Whelton PK. The impact of JNV VI guidelines on treatment recommendations in the US population. Hypertension 2002; 39:897–902.

24. Mancia G, Facchetti R, Bombelli M et al. Relationship of office, home and ambulatory blood pressure to blood glucose and lipid variables in the PAMELA population. Hypertension 2005; 45:1072–7.

25. Medical Research Council/British Heart Foundation Heart Protection Study of cholesterol lowering with simvastatin in 20536 high-risk individuals: a randomised placebo-controlled trial. Lancet 2002; 360:7–22.

26. Sever PS, Dahlof B, Poulter NR et al; ASCOT Investigators. Prevention of coronary and stroke events with atorvastatin in hypertensive patients who have average or lower-than-average cholesterol concentrations, in the Anglo-Scandinavian Cardiac Outcomes Trial – Lipid Lowering Arm (ASCOT-LLA): a multicentre randomised controlled trial. Lancet 2003; 361:1149–58.

27. Executive Summary of the Third Report of the National Cholesterol Education Program (NCEP) Expert Panel on Detection, Evaluation and Treatment of High Blood Cholesterol in Adults (Adult Treatment Panel III). JAMA 2001; 285:2486–97.

28. Grundy SM, Brewer HB Jr, Cleeman JI, Smith SC Jr, Lenfant C; National Heart, Lung, and Blood Institute; American Heart Association. Definition of metabolic syndrome: report of the National Heart, Lung, and Blood Institute/American Heart Association conference on scientific issues related to definition. Circulation 2004; 109:433–8.

29. Grassi G, Seravalle G, Dell'Oro R, et al. Comparative effects of candesartan and hydrochlorothiazide on blood pressure, insulin sensitivity and sympathetic drive in obese hypertensive individuals: results of the CROSS study. J Hypertens 2003; 21:1761–9.

30. Kurtz TW, Pravenec M. Antidiabetic mechanisms of angiotensin-converting enzyme inhibitors and angiotensin II receptor antagonists: beyond the renin–angiotensin system. J Hypertens 2004; 22:2253–61.

Angiotensin II antagonists and protection against subclinical cardiac and vascular damage

Enrico Agabiti-Rosei, Maria Lorenza Muiesan, and Damiano Rizzoni

8

Introduction

The renin–angiotensin system (RAS) is directly involved in blood pressure regulation as well as in the pathophysiology of hypertension by acting as an important stimulus to cardiovascular growth and remodeling. In addition, it has also been proposed that an elevated plasma renin activity might represent an independent risk factor for cardiovascular disease.[1]

The blockade of the RAS system by angiotensin converting enzyme (ACE) inhibitors has represented a significant advance in cardiovascular therapy, since it has facilitated control of both blood pressure and regression of cardiac and vascular hypertrophy. However, there are some limitations inherent to this approach, including the side effect of cough. As the pharmacologic effects of angiotensin are mediated by specific cell surface angiotensin receptors, the next logical development in the blockade of RAS was the production of orally active, specific angiotensin II receptor type 1 (AT$_1$) antagonists. There are theoretical grounds for supposing that AT$_1$ receptor antagonists could be even more effective than ACE inhibitors on structural abnormalities both in the heart and in the vessels. First, selective inhibition of AT$_1$ receptors is accompanied by an increase in circulating (and, probably, also in tissue) levels of angiotensin II. The raised angiotensin II levels will presumably cause increased stimulation of AT$_2$ receptors,[2] which could further inhibit smooth muscle cell growth and stimulate cellular apoptosis.[3] Secondly, in the heart and in the vessels, angiotensin II may be produced through chymase-dependent pathways, thus bypassing ACE inhibition;[2] therefore, direct inhibition of the AT_1 receptors may be more effective than ACE blockade in blocking the RAS activity. Although the mechanism of action is, roughly speaking, similar for the ACE inhibitors and the AT_1 antagonists, the two classes of drugs may present partially different actions on cardiovascular structure and a different incidence of side effects. In this chapter the available evidence on the protection against subclinical cardiac and vascular damage in hypertension by angiotensin II antagonists is reported and discussed.

Effects on cardiac damage

Left ventricular hypertrophy

Left ventricular hypertrophy (LVH) has been shown to be an independent risk factor for cardiovascular morbidity and mortality, including coronary artery disease, heart failure, stroke, and sudden death.[1–3] The increase in the relative risk for fatal events is doubled in patients with coronary artery disease and fourfold greater in patients with normal coronary arteries.[4,5] A linear and progressive relationship exists between LV mass and the risk of cardiovascular events.[3,6] LV mass regression is associated with an improvement in survival in hypertensive patients[7–10] and therefore regression of LVH represents a major goal of antihypertensive treatment.

Hypertensive heart disease involves a structural remodeling of cardiomyocytes and non-myocytes; fibroblasts contribute to the perivascular fibrosis that initially surrounds intramural coronary arteries and thereafter moves into the interstitial space.[11,12] The fibrosis consists of the increase of fibrillar collagen type I and type III and may be responsible for progressive abnormalities of diastolic ventricular filling and relaxation, of systolic function, and of cardiac rhythm and conduction, therefore contributing to the risk associated with LVH.[13] The excess of ventricular collagen may be the result of increased collagen synthesis, but also of insufficient collagen degradation by interstitial collagenase,[14] and, in particular, by metalloproteinase 1 (MMP-1), whose activity is regulated by specific tissue inhibitors of metalloproteinases (TIMP).[15]

Experimental studies have clarified the role of the renin–angiotensin–aldosterone system (RAAS) in mediating LVH. By stimulating the angiotensin receptor, angiotensin II induces hypertrophy and hyperplasia in myocytes and may regulate myofibroblast collagen synthesis. Excess angiotensin II production may regulate the expression of fibrogenic cytokine transforming growth factor-β_1 (TGF-β_1). Autocrine induction by TGF-β_1 of the genes coding for extracellular matrix proteins determines perivascular and interstitial fibrosis.

Angiotensin II may also regulate collagen degradation by reducing the activity of interstitial matrix MMP-1 activity in adult human cardiac fibroblasts and by enhancing the production of TIMP-1 (tissue inhibitor of metalloproteinase-1) in endothelial cells.

Angiotensin II stimulates TGF-β_1 gene expression, and promotes the conversion of latent TGF-β_1 into the active form.[16,17]

An increase in TGF-β_1 expression is also observed during LVH development in TGR(mRen2)27 (Ren2) rats, a monogenetic model of hypertension with low plasma and renal renin and high expression of renin in cardiac tissue.[18] The role of TGF-β_1 in the progression from compensated cardiac hypertrophy to cardiac dysfunction and heart failure is still not completely understood.

Angiotensin II may cause hypertrophy and favor fibrosis acting through other mechanisms, including the activation of myocardial calcineurin, which is reduced by blockade of AT_1 antagonists,[19] or the increase in intracellular calcium.[20]

Aldosterone may also stimulate extracellular collagen deposition and myocardial fibrosis.[21,22]

The pathogenic role of the RAAS in the development of human hypertensive LVH requires confirmation, although LV mass is significantly greater in renovascular hypertension and primary aldosteronism in comparison with essential hypertension.[23–25] There is also a correlation between LV mass and plasma aldosterone that is independent of blood pressure.[22]

The regression of structural remodeling in the hypertensive heart represents a goal of pharmacologic treatment, since a simple reduction in blood pressure in arterial hypertension may be unable to reduce fibroblast growth and collagen turnover. Therapeutic strategies have included the use of ACE inhibitors, AT_1 antagonists, endothelin A and B receptor antagonists, and aldosterone receptor antagonists. More recently, metalloproteinase activity modulators have been proposed.

Chronic treatment with losartan (an AT_1 antagonist) resulted in the normalization of collagen synthesis and reversal of LV fibrosis in spontaneously hypertensive rats (SHR).[26] The effect of angiotensin II blockade is independent from the hemodynamic changes and a non-hypotensive dose of the AT_1 antagonist blunted the expression of LV TGF- β_1, thus reducing collagen production and perivascular fibrosis in the hypertensive Ren2 rats.[18]

This effect, at least in part independent from blood pressure decrease, was also confirmed in a study[27] aimed at evaluating the effects on cardiac (and vascular) structure, including findings at the cellular level, of the ACE inhibitor enalapril and of the AT_1 antagonist losartan. SHR were treated from age 4 to 12 weeks with enalapril (25 mg/kg/day) or losartan (15 mg/kg/day). Untreated Wistar-Kyoto (WKY) and SHR were also studied. Rats were killed at 13 weeks, and the heart was weighed. Systolic blood pressure was significantly reduced by both drugs, but, with the doses of drugs chosen for this study, the hypotensive effect was greater with enalapril than with losartan. In the enalapril and losartan groups there were similar reductions in relative LV mass, despite the smaller hypotensive effect of the angiotensin II antagonist.

More recently, the effect on cardiac mass and structure of the ACE inhibitor enalapril and of the different AT_1 antagonists (losartan and olmesartan) were compared: all drugs reduced LV mass, although olmesartan and losartan were more effective than enalapril in reducing the collagen content in the heart and aorta.[27,28]

Several meta-analyses have clearly shown that not all classes of antihypertensive drugs have the same effect on LV mass.

The more recent meta-analysis[29] has included a large amount of data obtained from all randomized, controlled trials performed with angiotensin receptor blockers (6 studies, 9 arms of treatment, 248 patients). After adjustment for blood pressure and treatment duration, the decrease of LV mass was 13% with AT_1 antagonists, 10% with ACE inhibitors, 11% with calcium antagonists, 8% with diuretics, and 6% with β-blockers. The difference was statistically significant in a paired comparison between β-blockers and AT_1 antagonists, ACE inhibitors and calcium antagonists.

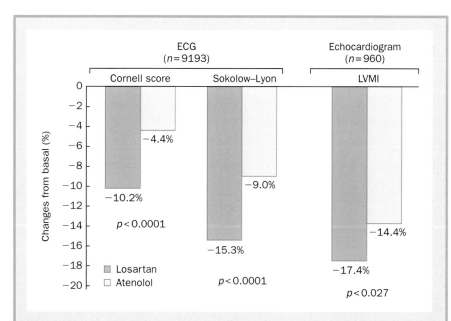

Figure 8.1

Effect of antihypertensive treatment on electrocardiographic (ECG) and echocardiographic indices of left ventricular hypertrophy (LVH) in the LIFE study. LVMI, left ventricular mass index. Modified from Dahlof et al[30] and Lindholm et al.[31]

The effect of angiotensin II antagonists on LVH regression has been compared with that of the β-blocker atenolol in two studies. The efficacy of angiotensin II antagonists was always greater than that of the β-blocker[30-32] (Figure 8.1). The Losartan Intervention For Endpoint reduction in hypertension (LIFE) trial was a large-scale trial that compared losartan-based and atenolol-based treatment in hypertensive patients with ECG-LVH.[32] The trial, after a mean period of follow-up of 4.8 years, has confirmed the true benefits of angiotensin II antagonists vs β-blockers, with a 13% reduction in the relative risk of composite end point (death, myocardial infarction, and stroke).[32] About one-third of the benefit was related to the greater regression of LVH obtained with losartan, and was clearly evident by both the analysis of ECG tracings,[33] and by the measurement of LV mass with the echocardiogram.[34] The effect of losartan-based treatment on LVH was independent of blood pressure reduction (similar in the two arms of treatment) and continuous over time.

The CATCH study was the only one to compare an ACE inhibitor-based and an angiotensin II antagonist-based treatment for 1 year in hypertensive patients.[35] For similar blood pressure reduction, the decrease in LV mass with candesartan was similar to that of the ACE inhibitor (-10.9% and -8.4% during treatment with enalapril or candesartan, respectively), although the proportion of patients achieving normalization of left ventricular mass index (LVMI) or changing from concentric to eccentric geometry of the left ventricle was higher with candesartan (Table 8.1).

Similar results have been obtained in a smaller group of hypertensive patients with diabetes mellitus type 2, treated for 1 year with enalapril or candesartan.[36]

It has been also suggested that gene polymorphisms of the RAAS are linked to hypertension and to hypertensive cardiac, vascular, and/or renal damage. The association between LVH and the ACE I/D polymorphism and both the M235T or the T174M polymorphisms of angiotensinogen have been studied extensively, with conflicting results.[37]

The aldosterone synthase (CYP11B2) 344T/C polymorphism was shown to be related to left ventricular structure (greater LV end-diastolic diameter and smaller relative wall thickness in hypertensive subjects with the CC genotype) in young hypertensive males[38] and in a general population,[39] possibly linked to elevated circulating aldosterone levels.

Moreover the AT$_2$-receptor 1675 G/A polymorphism and LVH have been also found to be associated, independently of blood pressure.[40] In the SILVHIA study (see Table 8.1), the association between several polymorphisms of the RAAS and changes in LVMI during antihypertensive treatment with an AT$_1$ receptor blocker or a β-blocker were assessed. The angiotensinogen T174M and M235T polymorphisms were related to the change in LVH during treatment with irbesartan, angiotensinogen T174M being the most powerful predictor of LV mass changes.[41]

Table 8.1
Changes in LV mass index (LVMI), relative wall thickness (RWT), and systolic blood pressure (SBP) in comparative studies with angiotensin II antagonists.

Study	Treatment	Number of patients	Change in LVMI	Change in RWT	Change in SBP (mmHg)
Thurmann et al[46]	Valsartan	29	$-21 g/m^2$*	-0.03	-17
	Atenolol	29	$-10 g/m^2$	-0.03	-14
Muller-Brunotte et al;[30] SILVHIA	Irbesartan	54	$-26 g/m^2$*	-0.06	-28
	Atenolol	58	$-14 g/m^2$	-0.05	-21
Dahlof et al;[31] REGAAL	Losartan	96	$-7 g/m^2$*	-0.01	-25
	Atenolol	87	$-3.7 g/m^2$	$+0.01$	-28*
Cuspidi et al;[35] CATCH	Candesartan	91	$-16 g/m^2$	-0.03	-28
	Enalapril	105	$-18 g/m^2$	-0.03	-26

*statistically significant

Effect on myocardial fibrosis

In consideration of the profibrotic effect of angiotensin II, it seems particularly interesting to evaluate the effect of antihypertensive treatment on the myocardial tissue composition, which possibly affects the fibrous perivascular and interstitial tissue. This hypothesis has been addressed in a study comparing the administration of an AT_1 antagonist or a dihydropyridinic calcium antagonist in essential hypertensive patients with LVH at baseline. Myocardial fibrosis, evaluated by measuring collagen content with intramyocardial biopsies, decreased significantly in the losartan-treated patients, and remained unchanged in the amlodipine-treated patients, despite no differences in blood pressure control.[42] The reduction in myocardial collagen content was paralleled by a significant decrease of transmitral early diastolic flow velocity deceleration time, suggesting an improvement of LV diastolic filling (Figure 8.2).

For obvious reasons myocardial collagen content cannot be routinely assessed by intramyocardial biopsies and it has become recently possible to evaluate abnormalities of myocardial tissue by ultrasound. In the REGAAL study (LVH REGression with the Angiotensin Antagonist Losartan) (see Table 8.1), echoreflectivity analysis was performed, according to changes in LV mass in 106 out of 225 hypertensive patients with LVH participating in the main study.[31] Despite similar antihypertensive effects, the reduction in LVMI was statistically significant in losartan-treated patients but not so in those treated with atenolol. Losartan reduced the videodensitometry broadband (a parameter shown to correlate with collagen content) after 36 weeks of treatment, whereas atenolol treatment was associated with an increase in broadband amplitude, suggesting that losartan may decrease myocardial collagen content, whereas atenolol does not.[43]

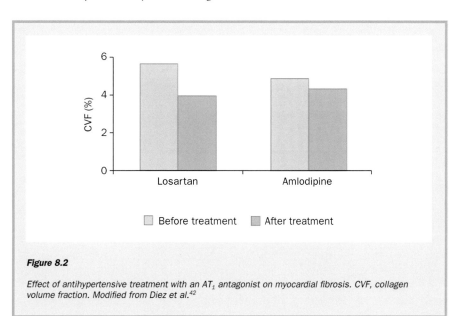

Figure 8.2

Effect of antihypertensive treatment with an AT_1 antagonist on myocardial fibrosis. CVF, collagen volume fraction. Modified from Diez et al.[42]

Effect on LV function

Diastolic dysfunction is common in hypertensive patients, mainly in those with hypertensive LV hypertrophy, even in the presence of normal LV systolic function or when asymptomatic LV systolic dysfunction has developed. The impairment of LV diastolic relaxation implies a worse prognosis for cardiovascular events, also independently of LV mass and blood pressure.[44] In addition, diastolic dysfunction may predict the subsequent development of clinically overt heart failure.[45]

Some studies have evaluated the effect of AT_1 receptor blockers on LV diastolic function, mainly by the measurement of transmitral flow and LV outflow tract velocities. In three studies, the therapy with valsartan,[46] candesartan,[35] or losartan[31] improved the E/A ratio only in some patients with hypertensive LVH.

On the contrary, two smaller studies were able to show an improvement in diastolic filling in patients without LVH after a few weeks of treatment with valsartan by radionuclide scintigraphy[47] and in patients with hypertensive heart disease by Doppler echocardiography.[48]

A very recent analysis[49] of the SILVHIA (Swedish Irbesartan Left Ventricular Hypertrophy Investigation versus Atenolol) study has shown that the AT_1 receptor blocker irbesartan significantly improves diastolic function to the same extent as atenolol in patients with cardiac hypertrophy, although this improvement may be shown only when several echocardiographic measures of diastolic function are taken into consideration (the E/A ratio of transmitral flow, the E wave deceleration time, S/D ratio of pulmonary veins flow, the isovolumic relaxation time, and ratio of the magnitude of motion due to atrial systole to the total diastolic atrioventricular plane displacement).

The use of angiotensin II antagonists may be particularly beneficial not only in patients with Langerhans cell histiocytosis (LCH) and/or LV dysfunction, but also in those with LV diastolic failure, as suggested by the results of the 'Preserved' arm of the CHARM (Candesartan in Heart failure Assessment of Reduction in Mortality and morbidity program) study.[50] The effect of candesartan, as compared to placebo (conventional therapy), was evaluated in 3023 patients with heart failure (NYHA class II–IV) and LV ejection fraction within normal limits. During a follow-up of 36 months, a lower rate of hospitalization for heart failure was observed in patients randomized to candesartan (hazard ratio = 0.84, 95% CI = 0.70–1.00), suggesting a potential benefit of angiotensin II antagonist treatment in addition to conventional treatment.

Effect on large vessels

Recent interest has focused on the role of angiotensin II, acting via the AT_1 receptor, in the development of vascular disease.[51] Most of the known vascular actions of angiotensin II are mediated by the angiotensin type-1 receptor, and AT_1 receptor blockers have been widely used as antihypertensive drugs, with the perspective of a vascular protective action.

Three studies have given useful information on the effect of chronic treatment with AT_1 antagonists on carotid artery morphology, as evaluated by non-invasive echo Doppler techniques; these studies, comprising a relatively small number of patients, have shown a lower thickness of intima-media during treatment with angiotensin II antagonists in respect with patients treated with β-blockers.[52,53] When losartan was compared with an ACE inhibitor, the latter was more effective in reducing intima-media thickness after 1 year of treatment.[54]

An ongoing study (Multicenter Olmesartan atherosclerosis Regression Evaluation; MORE) will give a more precise assessment of the effect of long-term treatment with an AT_1 receptor antagonist (olmesartan) and with a β-blocker (atenolol) on carotid atherosclerosis, even with the use of the non-invasive 3D plaque measurement.

Another study (the Candesartan Atenolol Carotid Haemodynamic Endpoint Trial, CACHET) is actually ongoing with the aim of comparing the effects of two antihypertensive regimens, based either on a β-blocker or on an angiotensin receptor blocker, on carotid intima-media thickness, and to evaluate the effects of these antihypertensive regimens on local fluid dynamics.[55]

Arterial stiffness represents a parameter of vascular structure and function that increases in the presence of several risk factors, including hypertension and end-stage renal disease, and that may be influenced by the activation of the RAAS. Measures of arterial compliance are associated with an increased risk of total and cardiovascular mortality and an improvement of arterial stiffness, and may represent an additional target for antihypertensive treatment.[56,57]

Two small studies have evaluated the effects of the treatment with angiotensin AT_1 receptor blocker (losartan) in comparison to that with hydrochlorothiazide or with placebo, on arterial compliance, measured by carotido-femoral pulse-wave velocity.[58,59] One more recent study has also analyzed the effect of antihypertensive treatment for 6 weeks with valsartan or hydrochlorothiazide or placebo on the augmentation index, i.e. a parameter that gives an estimate of the central aortic pressure augmentation due to the reflected pressure wave. The results of this study have shown that valsartan, but not the diuretic, reduced the augmentation index, and this effect was independent of supine blood pressure measurements.[60] The possibility of improving arterial compliance and decreasing the reflected wave central augmentation index by the use of angiotensin II antagonists may contribute to the prevention and/or regression of LVH in hypertensive patients.

Effects on small resistance artery

The RAS seems to play a key role in the development of vascular structural alterations that are usually observed both in humans and in animal models of genetic or experimental hypertension.[61,62] In fact, in patients with activation of the RAAS, such as those with renovascular hypertension and primary aldosteronism, particularly pronounced alterations in subcutaneous small resistance artery structure were observed, as indicated by a very marked increase of the tunica media to internal lumen ratio.[24,63]

Whereas in essential hypertension the major part of the structural changes observed in small arteries is the consequence of eutrophic remodeling (rearrangement of the same amount of wall material around a narrowed lumen),[64] without net cell growth, in patients with renovascular hypertension, a more evident contribution of cell growth, leading to the development of hypertrophic remodeling (vascular smooth muscle cell hypertrophy or hyperplasia), may be observed.[24,63] It has also been previously demonstrated that hypertrophic remodeling of subcutaneous small arteries in renovascular hypertension may be selectively ascribed to vascular smooth muscle cell hypertrophy.[63] In addition, in patients with renovascular hypertension or primary aldosteronism, close correlations between small resistance artery structure and cardiac or carotid artery structure may be observed,[24] thus suggesting that the RAS may act as a 'synchronizer' of the cardiovascular structure, by stimulating smooth muscle cell remodeling at the same time at both the cardiac and the vascular level.

Structural alterations of the microcirculation are involved in the mechanisms which determine blood pressure,[62] since they may amplify the effect of any hypertensive stimulus.[65] In addition, they play a significant role in reducing organ flow reserve,[66] and are probably the most potent predictor of cardiovascular events in high-risk hypertensive patients.[67]

To the extent that circulating or tissue RAAS may play a relevant role in the development of structural alterations in the microcirculation, drugs that can reduce RAAS activity could be particularly advantageous in terms of regression of such abnormalities.

Data in animal models of genetic hypertension

Like ACE inhibitors,[68–73] AT$_1$ antagonists may cause regression of vascular structural alterations[74–76] in SHR. Ledingham and Laverty[77] have demonstrated a relevant beneficial effect of the angiotensin II receptor antagonist valsartan on structural alterations in mesenteric small resistance arteries of New Zealand genetically hypertensive rats, using a stereologic method. However, New Zealand hypertensive rats showed the presence of hypertrophic remodeling. On the contrary, in mesenteric arteries of SHR, an inward eutrophic remodeling[78] was observed, the same pattern of structural alterations that may be detected in human essential hypertension.[79] We have recently performed some studies aimed at evaluating the effects on vascular structure of the ACE inhibitor enalapril and of the AT$_1$ antagonists candesartan,[79] losartan,[80] and olmesartan.[28] The ACE inhibitor and the AT$_1$ antagonists were significantly and equally effective in inducing a reduction of structural alterations in mesenteric small resistance arteries. However, the AT$_1$ antagonists olmesartan and losartan were more effective than enalapril in preventing alterations of aortic and cardiac extracellular matrix,[27,28] respectively.

Data in human hypertension

In the last few years some studies have demonstrated a significant reduction[81,82] and – in some cases – an almost complete normalization of structural alterations in human subcutaneous small resistance arteries after long-term therapy with ACE inhibitors.[83–86] The AT$_1$ antagonist losartan, given for 1 year to essential hypertensive patients, was able to completely normalize small resistance artery structure, whereas the β-blocker atenolol had no effect despite a similar blood pressure reduction.[87] Those patients who did not respond to the β-blocker were subsequently treated with a different AT$_1$ antagonist, irbesartan, and a normalization of vascular structure was then observed.[88] Therefore, AT$_1$ antagonists seem to be very effective in normalizing structural alterations in the microcirculation. However, no direct comparison between ACE inhibitors and AT$_1$ antagonists in patients with essential hypertension is presently available. On the other hand, a study directly comparing an ACE inhibitor, enalapril, and an AT$_1$ antagonist, candesartan, in diebetic hypertensive patients has been recently published.[36] The two drugs were equally effective in improving vascular structure; however, candesartan was more effective than enalapril

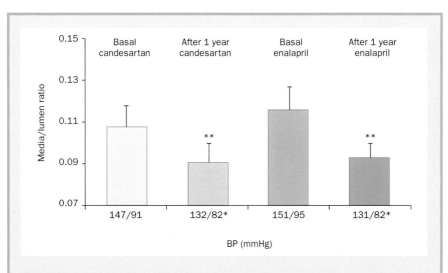

Figure 8.3

Effects of 1-year treatment with candesartan or enalapril on subcutaneous small resistance artery structure in diabetic hypertensive patients.[36]
**p<0.01 vs basal

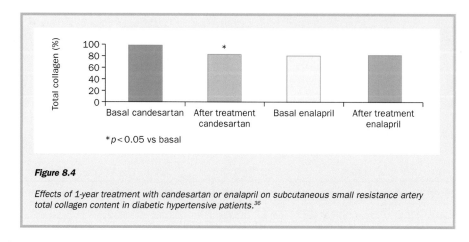

Figure 8.4

Effects of 1-year treatment with candesartan or enalapril on subcutaneous small resistance artery total collagen content in diabetic hypertensive patients.[36]

in reducing collagen content within the vascular walls (Figures 8.3 and 8.4). Therefore, the antifibrotic effect of the AT_1 antagonist seems to be more pronounced than that of an ACE inhibitor.

In the last two years, some studies have demonstrated that drugs that inhibit the RAAS (such as losartan, perindopril, and ramipril) may have some advantage, over other drugs, or beyond the decrease in blood pressure, in reducing morbidity and mortality in high-risk hypertensive patients. It is possible that their favorable effect on small resistance artery structure may at least in part explain the additional benefits. However it should be emphasized that the prognostic impact of the regression of vascular structural alterations per se is still unknown, and prospective studies are needed in order to clarify whether structural alterations in small resistance arteries may be considered an intermediate end point in the evaluation of the effects of antihypertensive treatment.

Conclusions

AT_1 antagonists represent a new class of antihypertensive drugs with promising characteristics. They may possess some advantages over the ACE inhibitors, but this aspect is presently under evaluation, and we should wait for consistent data, which will be obtained from several large prospective studies that are presently in progress.

References

1.   Levy D, Anderson KM, Savage DD et al. Echocardiographically detected left ventricular hypertrophy: prevalence and risk factors. The Framingham Heart Study. Ann Intern Med 1988; 108:7–13.
2.   Casale PN, Devereux RB, Milner M et al. Value of echocardiographic measurement of left ventricular mass in predicting cardiovascular morbid events in hypertensive men. Ann Intern Med 1986; 105:173–8.

3. Levy D, Garrison RJ, Savage DD, Kannel WB, Castelli WP. Prognostic implications of echocardiographically determined left ventricular mass in the Framingham Heart Study. N Engl J Med 1990; 322:1561–6.

4. Cooper RS, Simmons BE, Castaner A et al. Left ventricular hypertrophy is associated with worse survival independent of ventricular function and number of coronary arteries severely narrowed. Am J Cardiol 1990; 65:441–5.

5. Ghali JK, Liao Y, Simmons B et al. The prognostic role of left ventricular hypertrophy in patients with or without coronary artery disease. Ann Intern Med 1992; 117:831–6.

6. Schillaci G, Verdecchia P, Porcellati C et al. Continuous relation between left ventricular mass and cardiovascular risk in essential hypertension. Hypertension 2000; 35:580–6.

7. Muiesan ML, Salvetti M, Rizzoni D et al. Association of change in left ventricular mass with prognosis during long-term antihypertensive treatment. J Hypertens 1995; 13:1091–7.

8. Verdecchia P, Schillaci G, Borgioni I et al. Prognostic significance of serial changes in left ventricular mass in essential hypertension. Circulation 1998; 97:48–54.

9. Koren MJ, Ulin RJ, Koren AT, Laragh JH, Devereux RB. Left ventricular mass changes during treatment and outcome in patients with essential hypertension. Am J Hypertens 2002; 15:1021–8.

10. Devereux RB, Wachtell K, Gerdts E et al. Prognostic significance of left ventricular mass change during treatment of hypertension. JAMA 2004; 292:2350–6.

11. Weber KT, Brilla CG. Pathological hypertrophy and cardiac interstitium: fibrosis and renin–angiotensin–aldosterone system. Circulation 1991; 83:1849–53.

12. Brilla CG, Zhou G, Matsubara L, Weber KT. Collagen metabolism in cultured adult rat cardiac fibroblasts: response to angiotensin II and aldosterone. J Mol Cell Cardiol 1994; 26:809–20.

13. Frohlich E. Risk mechanisms in hypertensive heart disease. Hypertension 1999; 34(Part 2):782–9.

14. Woessner JF. Matrix metalloproteinases and their inhibitors in connective tissue remodeling. FASEB J 1991; 5:2145–54.

15. Weber KT. Collagen matrix synthesis and degradation in the development and regression of left ventricular hypertrophy. Cardiovasc Rev Rep 1991; 12:61–9.

16. Pathak M, Sarkar S, Vellaichamy E, Sen S. Role of myocytes in myocardial collagen production. Hypertension 2001; 37:833–40.

17. Schultz Jel J, Witt SA, Glascock BJ et al. TGF β1 mediates the hypertrophic cardiomyocyte growth induced by angiotensin II. J Clin Invest 2002; 109:787–96.

18. Pinto Y, Pinto-Sietsma SJ, Philipp T et al. Reduction in left ventricular messenger RNA for transforming growth factor β1 attenuates left ventricular fibrosis and improves survival without lowering blood pressure in the hypertensive TGR(mRen2)27 rat. Circulation 2000; 36:747–54.

19. Nagata K, Somura F, Obata K et al. AT1 receptor blockade reduces cardiac calcineurin activity in hypertensive rats. Hypertension 2002; 40:168–74.

20. Ostrom RS, Naugle JE, Hase M et al. Angiotensin II enhances adenylyl cyclase signaling via Ca^{2+}/calmodulin. Gq-Gs cross-talk regulates collagen production in cardiac fibroblasts. J Biol Chem 2003; 278:24461–8.

21. Duprez D, Bauwens F, De Buyzere ML et al. Influence of arterial blood pressure and aldosterone on left ventricular hypertrophy in moderate essential hypertension. Am J Cardiol 1993; 71:17A–20A.

22. Schlaich MP, Schobel HP, Hilgers K, Schmieder RE. Impact of aldosterone on left ventricular structure and function in young normotensive and mildly hypertensive subjects. Am J Cardiol 2000; 85:1199–206.

23. Losito A, Faguli RM, Zampi I et al. Comparison of target organ damage in renovascular and essential hypertension. Am J Hypertens 1996; 9:1062–7.

24. Rizzoni D, Muiesan ML, Porteri E et al. Relations between cardiac and vascular structure in patients with primary and secondary hypertension. J Am Coll Cardiol 1998; 32(4):985–92.

25. Rossi GP, Sacchetto A, Pavan E et al. Remodeling of the left ventricle in primary aldosteronism due to Conn's adenoma. Circulation 1997; 95:1471–8.

26. Varo N, Iraburu MJ, Varela M et al. Chronic AT1 blockade stimulates extracellular collagen type 1 degradation and reverses myocardial fibrosis in spontaneously hypertensive rats. Hypertension 2000; 35:1197–1202.

27. Rizzoni D, Rodella L, Porteri E et al. Effects of losartan and enalapril at different doses on cardiac and renal interstitial matrix in spontaneously hypertensive rats. Clin Exp Hypertens 2003; 25(7):427–41.

28. Porteri E, Rodella L, Rizzoni D et al. Effects of olmesartan and enalapril at low or high doses on cardiac, renal and vascular interstitial matrix in spontaneously hypertensive rats. Blood Press 2005; 14:184–92.

29. Klingbeil AU, Schneider M, Martus P, Messerli FH, Schmieder RE. A meta-analysis of the effects of treatment on left ventricular mass in essential hypertension. Am J Med 2003; 115:41–6.

30. Malmqvist K, Kahan T, Edner M et al. Regression of left ventricular hypertrophy in human hypertension with irbesartan. J Hypertens 2001; 19:1167–76.

31. Dahlof B, Zanchetti A, Diez J et al, for the REGAAL Study Investigators. Effects of losartan and atenolol on left ventricular mass and neurohormonal profile in patients with essential hypertension and left ventricular hypertrophy. J Hypertens 2002; 20:1855–64.

32. Lindholm LH, Ibsen H, Dahlöf B et al, LIFE Study Group. Cardiovascular morbidity and mortality in the Losartan Intervention For Endpoint reduction in hypertension study (LIFE): a randomised trial against atenolol. Lancet 2002; 359:995–1003.

33. Okin PM, Devereux RB, Jern S et al. Losartan Intervention For Endpoint reduction in hypertension (LIFE) Study Investigators. Regression of electrocardiographic left ventricular hypertrophy by losartan versus atenolol. The Losartan Intervention For Endpoint reduction in hypertension (LIFE) study. Circulation 2003; 108:684–90.

34. Devereux RB, Dahlöf B, Gerdts E et al. Regression of hypertensive left ventricular hypertrophy by losartan compared with atenolol: the Losartan Intervention For Endpoint reduction in hypertension (LIFE) trial. Circulation 2004; 110:1456–62.

35. Cuspidi C, Muiesan ML, Valagussa L et al; CATCH investigators. Comparative effects of candesartan and enalapril on left ventricular hypertrophy in patients with essential hypertension: the candesartan assessment in the treatment of cardiac hypertrophy (CATCH) study. J Hypertens 2002; 20:2293–300.

36. Rizzoni D, Porteri E, De Ciuceis C et al. Effects of treatment with candesartan or enalapril on subcutaneous small resistance artery structure in hypertensive patients with NIDDM. Hypertension 2005; 45(Part 2):659–65.

37. Danser AH, Schunkert H. Renin–angiotensin system gene polymorphisms: potential mechanisms for their association with cardiovascular diseases. Eur J Pharmacol 2000; 410:303–16.

38. Delles C, Erdmann J, Jacobi J et al. Aldosterone synthase (CYP11B2)-344C/T polymorphism is associated with left ventricular structure in human arterial hypertension. J Am Coll Cardiol 2001; 37:878–84.

39. Castellano M, Rossi F, Rivadossi F et al. Aldosterone synthase gene polymorphism and cardiovascular phenotypes in a general population. J Hypertens 2000; 18(Suppl 4):174.

40. Schmieder RE, Erdmann J, Delles C et al. Effects of angiotensin II type-2 receptor gene 1675 G/A on left ventricular structure in humans. J Am Coll Cardiol 2001; 37:175–82.

41. Kurland L, Melhus H, Karlsson J et al. Polymorphisms in the angiotensinogen and angiotensin II type 1 receptor gene are related to change in left ventricular mass during antihypertensive treatment: results from the Swedish Irbesartan Left Ventricular Hypertrophy Investigation versus Atenolol (SILVHIA) Trial. J Hypertens 2002; 20:657–63.

42. Diez J, Querejeta R, Lopez B et al. Losartan-dependent regression of myocardial fibrosis is associated with reduction of left ventricular chamber stiffness in hypertensive patients. Circulation 2002; 105:2512–17.

43. Ciulla M, Paliotti R, Esposito A et al. Different effects of antihypertensive therapies based on losartan or atenolol on ultrasound and biochemical markers of myocardial fibrosis. Results of a randomized trial. Circulation 2004; 110:552–7.

44. Schillaci G, Pasqualini L, Verdecchia P et al. Prognostic significance of left ventricular diastolic dysfunction in essential hypertension. J Am Coll Cardiol 2002; 39:2005–11.

45. Aurigemma GP, Gottdiener JS, Shemanski L, Gardin J, Kitzman D. Predictive value of systolic and diastolic function for incident congestive heart failure in the elderly: the cardiovascular health study. J Am Coll Cardiol 2001; 37:1042–8.

46. Thürmann PA, Kenedi P, Schmidt A, Harder S, Rietbrock N. Influence of the angiotensin II

antagonist valsartan on left ventricular hypertrophy in patients with essential hypertension. Circulation 1998; 98:2037–41.

47. Cuocolo A, Storto G, Izzo R et al. Effects of valsartan on left ventricular diastolic function in patients with mild or moderate essential hypertension: comparison with enalapril. J Hypertens 1999; 17:1759–66.

48. Isobe N, Taniguchi K, Oshima S et al. Candesartan cilexetil improves left ventricular function, left ventricular hypertrophy, and endothelial function in patients with hypertensive heart disease. Circ J 2002; 66:993–9.

49. Muller-Brunotte R, Edner M, Malmqvist K, Kahan T. Irbesartan and atenolol improve diastolic function in patients with hypertensive left ventricular hypertrophy. J Hypertens 2005; 23:633–40.

50. Yusuf S, Pfeffer MA, Swedberg K et al, for the CHARM Investigators and Committees. Effects of candesartan in patients with chronic heart failure and preserved left ventricular systolic function: the CHARM-Preserved Trial. Lancet 2003; 362:777–81.

51. Drexler H, Schieffer B. Angiotensin II and atherosclerosis. In: Unger T, Scholkens B, eds. Angiotensin. Berlin: Springer-Verlag; 2004: Vol II, pp 21–39.

52. Ludwig M, Stapff M, Ribeiro A et al. Comparison of the effects of losartan and atenolol on common carotid artery intima-media thickness in patients with hypertension: results of a 2-year, double-blind, randomized, controlled study. Clin Ther 2002; 24(7):1175–93.

53. Olsen MH, Wachtell K, Neland K et al. Losartan but not atenolol reduce carotid artery hypertrophy in essential hypertension. A LIFE substudy. Blood Press 2005; 14(3):177–83.

54. Uchiyama-Tanaka Y, Mori Y, Kishimoto N et al. Comparison of the effects of quinapril and losartan on carotid artery intima-media thickness in patients with mild-to-moderate arterial hypertension. Kidney Blood Press Res 2005; 28(2):111–16.

55. Ariff B, Stanton A, Barratt D et al. Comparison of the effects of antihypertensive treatment with angiotensin II blockade and beta-blockade on carotid wall structure and haemodynamics: protocol and baseline demographics. J Renin Angiotensin Aldosterone Syst 2002; 3:116–22.

56. Blacher J, Asmar R, Djane S, London GM, Safar ME. Aortic pulse wave velocity as a marker of cardiovascular risk in hypertensive patients. Hypertension 1999; 33:1111–17.

57. Laurent S. Arterial stiffness: intermediate or surrogate endpoint for cardiovascular events? Eur Heart J 2005; 26:1252.

58. Klemsal TO, Moan A, Kjeldsen S. Effects of selective angiotensin II type 1 receptor blockade with losartan on arterial compliance in patients with mild essential hypertension. Blood Press 1999; 8:214–19.

59. Mahmud A, Feely J. Effect of angiotensin II receptor blockade on arterial stiffness: beyond blood pressure reduction. Am J Hypertens 2002; 15:1092–5.

60. Klingbeil A, John S, Schneider M et al. AT-1 receptor blockade improves augmentation index: a double-blind, randomized, controlled study. J Hypertens 2002; 20:2423–8.

61. Mulvany MJ. Resistance vessel growth and remodelling: cause or consequence in cardiovascular disease. J Human Hypertens 1995; 9:479–85.

62. Mulvany MJ. Small artery remodeling and significance in the development of hypertension. News Physiol Sci 2002; 17:105–9.

63. Rizzoni D, Porteri E, Castellano M et al. Vascular hypertrophy and remodeling in secondary hypertension. Hypertension 1996; 28:785–90.

64. Rizzoni D, Porteri E, Guelfi D et al. Cellular hypertrophy in subcutaneous small arteries of patients with renovascular hypertension. Hypertension 2000; 35:931–5.

65. Lever AF. Slow pressor mechanisms in hypertension: a role for hypertrophy of resistance vessels? J Hypertens 1986; 4:515–24.

66. Rizzoni D, Palombo C, Porteri E et al. Relationships between coronary vasodilator capacity and small artery remodeling in hypertensive patients. J Hypertens 2003; 21:625–32.

67. Rizzoni D, Porteri E, Boari GEM et al. Prognostic significance of small artery structure in hypertension. Circulation 2003; 108:2230–5.

68. Rizzoni D, Castellano M, Porteri E et al. Effects of low and high doses of fosinopril on the structure and function of resistance arteries. Hypertension 1995; 26:118–23.

69. Christensen KL, Jespersen LT, Mulvany MJ. Development of blood pressure in spontaneously

hypertensive rats after withdrawal of long-term treatment related to vascular structure. J Hypertens 1989; 7:83–90.

70. Harrap SB, Van der Merwe WM, Griffin SA, MacPherson F, Lever AF. Brief angiotensin converting enzyme inhibitor treatment in young spontaneously hypertensive rats reduces blood pressure long term. Hypertension 1990; 16:603–14.

71. Adams MA, Bobik A, Korner PI. Enalapril can prevent vascular amplifier development in spontaneously hypertensive rats. Hypertension 1990; 16:252–60.

72. Rizzoni D, Castellano M, Porteri E et al. Prolonged effects of short-term forsinopril on blood pressure and vascular morphology and function in rats. Am J Hypertens 1997; 10:1034–43.

73. Gibbons GH. Angiotensin-converting enzyme inhibition and vascular structure in hypertension. J Cardiovasc Pharmacol 1991; 18(Suppl 7):S19–24.

74. Li JS, Sharafi AM, Schiffrin EL. Effect of AT1 angiotensin-receptor blockade on structure and function of small resistance arteries in SHR. J Cardiovasc Pharmacol 1997; 30:75–83.

75. Morton JJ, Beattie EC, MacPherson F. Angiotensin II receptor antagonist losartan has persistent effect on blood pressure in the young spontaneously hypertensive rat: lack of relation to vascular structure. J Vasc Res 1992; 29:264–9.

76. Shaw LM, George PR, Oldham AA, Heagerty AM. A comparison of the effect of angiotensin converting enzyme inhibition and angiotensin II receptor antagonism on structural changes associated with hypertension in rat small arteries. J Hypertens 1995; 13:1135–43.

77. Ledingham JM, Laverty R. Remodelling of resistance arteries in genetically hypertensive rats by treatment with valsartan, an angiotensin II receptor antagonist. Clin Exp Pharmacol Physiol 1996; 23:576–8.

78. Heagerty AM, Aalkjaaer C, Bund SJ, Korsgaard N, Mulvany MJ. Small artery structure in hypertension. Dual process of remodeling and growth. Hypertension 1993; 21:391–7.

79. Rizzoni D, Porteri E, Piccoli A et al. Effects of candesartan cilexetil and enalapril on structural alterations and endothelial function in small resistance arteries of spontaneously hypertensive rats. J Cardiovasc Pharmacol 1998; 32:798–806.

80. Rizzoni D, Porteri E, Piccoli A et al. Effects of losartan and enalapril on small artery structure in hypertensive rats. Hypertension 1998; 32:305–10.

81. Rizzoni D, Muiesan ML, Porteri E et al. Effect of long-term antihypertensive treatment with lisinopril on resistance arteries in hypertensive patients with left ventricular hypertrophy. J Hypertens 1997; 15:197–204.

82. Thürmann PA, Stephens N, Heagerty AM et al. Influence of isradipine and spirapril on left ventricular hypertrophy and resistance arteries. Hypertension 1996; 28:450–6.

83. Schiffrin EL, Deng LY, Larochelle P. Effects of a β-blocker or a converting enzyme inhibitor on resistance arteries in essential hypertension. Hypertension 1994; 23:83–91.

84. Thybo NK, Stephens N, Cooper A et al. Effect of antihypertensive treatment on small arteries of patients with previously untreated essential hypertension. Hypertension 1995; 25(Part 1):474–81.

85. Sihm I, Schroeder AP, Aalkjaer C et al. Normalization of resistance artery structure and left ventricular morphology with a perindopril-based regimen. Can J Cardiol 1994; 10(Suppl D):30–2D.

86. Schiffrin EL, Deng LY. Comparison of effects of angiotensin I-converting enzyme inhibition and β-blockade for 2 years on function of small arteries from hypertensive patients. Hypertension 1995; 25(Part 2):699–703.

87. Schiffrin EL, Park JB, Intengan HD, Touyz RM. Correction of arterial structure and endothelial dysfunction in human essential hypertension by the angiotensin receptor antagonist losartan. Circulation 2000; 101:1653–9.

88. Schiffrin EL, Park JB, Pu Q. Effect of crossing over hypertensive patients from a beta-blocker to an angiotensin receptor antagonist on resistance artery structure and on endothelial function. J Hypertens 2002; 20:71–8.

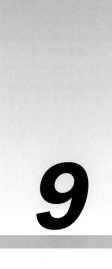

Angiotensin receptor blockers for chronic heart failure

John GF Cleland and Huan Loh

Introduction

Angiotensin receptor blockers (ARBs) are widely used for the management of patients with heart failure. Improving symptoms and quality of life, reducing morbidity and disability, and prolonging life are the key markers for efficacy of interventions for heart failure. Safety and tolerability are also of concern, but only if efficacy is proven first. The purpose of this chapter is to review the evidence that ARBs are effective in the above terms when used for the management of heart failure.

Most of the evidence for the clinical role of ARBs in the management of patients with major cardiac dysfunction has been obtained from seven (ELITE, ELITE II, RESOLVD, Val-HeFT, CHARM-alternative, CHARM-added, and CHARM-preserved) major trials of heart failure,[1–22] two meta-analyses of smaller trials (one of losartan[23] and the other of candesartan[24]), and two trials in the post-infarction setting (OPTIMAAL[25,26] and VALIANT[27,28]). Altogether, more than 30 000 patients have been included in these randomized controlled trials. A further trial investigating the role of an ARB in patients with heart failure and preserved LVSD (I-PRESERVE) and another comparing 50 mg vs 150 mg of losartan (HEAL) will not report for some years. Undoubtedly, more trials will follow.

Rationale for the use of ARBs in heart failure

The organization of the renin–angiotensin–aldosterone system (RAAS) is outlined in Figure 9.1. Angiotensin converting enzyme (ACE) is responsible not only for the production of angiotensin II (AII) but also for the degradation of bradykinin.[29,30] Other possible substrates for ACE include erythropoietin and the enkephalins.

Angiotensin II has numerous actions. The acute effects of AII include arterial and, probably, venous constriction, reduced parasympathetic and increased sympathetic nervous activity and, possibly, direct effects on the kidney, resulting in salt and water retention.[31–37] Chronic effects include cardiac and vascular remodeling and a potential role in the genesis of atheroma.[38,39]

Less is known about bradykinin because it is difficult to measure accurately, it acts very close to its site of synthesis with little spill-over into the circulation, and because pharmacologic tools for manipulating its actions on its receptor site have only recently become available.[29] In general, the actions of bradykinin are opposite to those of AII and include vasodilation and stimulation of nitric oxide and vasodilator prostaglandin production, the latter being a potential mechanism for the interaction between ACE inhibitors and aspirin.[29] Bradykinin may also have favorable effects on left ventricular remodeling, endothelial function, and the development of atheroma. However, bradykinin has also been purported to activate the sympathetic nervous system, a potentially undesirable effect,[40] and may be responsible for ACE inhibitor-induced cough and angioneurotic edema.

There are alternative pathways for the generation of AII. Chymase can convert angiotensin I to II by an ACE-independent pathway.[41–43] Whether it is present in sufficient quantity to generate

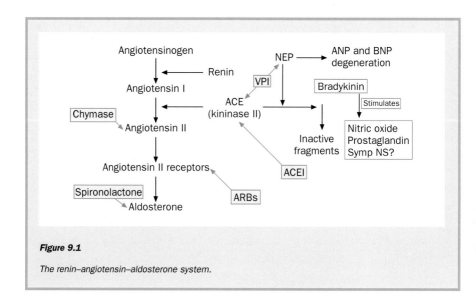

Figure 9.1

The renin–angiotensin–aldosterone system.

significant amounts of AII either systemically or at a local (tissue) level in humans is uncertain. Chymotrypsin, angiotensin-generating enzyme, and cathepsin D are other pathways for AII production that are not blocked by ACE inhibitors.

The current principal classification of angiotensin receptors in humans is into AT_1 and AT_2 receptors, but it is likely that the number of receptor subtypes described will increase. AT_1 receptors are widely distributed in the heart, on the luminal surface of the vascular endothelium, noradrenergic nerve terminals, adrenal cortex, and kidneys.[44,45] AT_2 receptor expression is high in fetal tissues and in healing wounds. In the human heart the AT_2 receptor predominates and the concentration is maintained or increased, compared with that of AT_1 receptors as chronic heart failure (CHF) develops.[46–48]

The AT_1 receptor appears responsible for the mediation of all the classical effects of AII.[41,42] Stimulation of the AT_2 receptor may cause vasodilation and have beneficial antiproliferative effects but may also stimulate apoptosis, which could have adverse effects on cardiovascular remodeling.[49,50] Thus, the clinical effects of selective AT_1 receptor blockade could be superior, inferior, or identical to those of non-selective AT receptor blockade.

Why might the effects of ARBs and ACE inhibitors differ?

ACE 'breakthrough'

Although acute administration of an ACE inhibitor reduces plasma AII to around the limit of detection, plasma AII (even when technically robust sampling and assay methods are used) and aldosterone are often not suppressed after several months of treatment.[51,52] Poor compliance might be responsible in some instances for the apparent loss of ACE inhibition but the problem appears too prevalent to be accounted for by poor compliance alone.[53] ACE inhibition leads to an accumulation of the precursor for AII, angiotensin I. Although 80% ACE inhibition may be enough to suppress AII formation at normal levels of angiotensin I, much more intense inhibition may be required in the presence of increased substrate. Small doses (e.g. 5 mg of enalapril or lisinopril) of an ACE inhibitor may be adequate to suppress AII initially, but much larger doses (e.g. 35 mg lisinopril or 40 mg enalapril) may be required for long-term inhibition. Increasing levels of angiotensin I may also be converted to AII through ACE-independent pathways and therefore even intense ACE inhibition may not be adequate to suppress AII production in the long term.[41–43] ARBs block the downstream effects of AII and therefore it does not matter which route generates AII.

AT_2 receptor stimulation

Activation of the RAAS is normally limited by negative feedback of AII on the AT_1 receptor. ARBs block the AT_1 receptor and therefore release the RAAS from negative feedback.

Accordingly, plasma concentrations of AII rise and, consequently, stimulation of the unblocked AT_2 receptor may increase. Therefore, unlike ACE inhibitors, ARBs may increase stimulation of the AT_2 receptor, which may or may not be beneficial (see above).

Bradykinin–prostaglandin and other pathways

ACE inhibitors, unlike ARBs, increase bradykinin[29] and hence nitric oxide and vasodilator and antiaggregatory prostaglandins. This could confer additional vasodilator, antithrombotic, and antiatherogenic effects on ACE inhibitors as well as having favorable effects on cardiovascular remodeling. Neutralization of the prostaglandin-mediated effects of ACE inhibition could account for the adverse interaction between aspirin and ACE inhibitors.[54–60] The lack of effect of ARBs on the bradykinin-prostaglandin pathway suggests that they might not reduce vascular events, especially coronary events, as effectively as ACE inhibitors. Although no adverse interaction between ARBs and aspirin would be expected, this reflects the lack of a beneficial ancillary effect of ARBs on prostaglandin metabolism.

ACE inhibitors may also inhibit other enzymes that could have beneficial (e.g. neutral endopeptidase or matrix metalloproteinases) or possibly deleterious effects on symptoms or cardiovascular remodeling.

Effects on hematocrit

ACE inhibitors cause hematocrit to fall, either because of hemodilution or because of a fall in red cell volume due to a decline in erythropoietin, an effect either mediated directly or through an improvement in renal blood flow.[37,61] Hemodilution could reduce oxygen uptake and transport and detract from the benefits of ACE inhibitors on symptoms and functional capacity. However, reducing hematocrit could also reduce the risk of thrombotic events. ARBs also reduce hematocrit.[16,62]

Electrophysiologic and autonomic effects

Compared to captopril, losartan may exert a greater effect on progressive electrical remodeling and QT dispersion.[63] However, ARBs (losartan 50 mg/day), unlike ACE inhibitors,[32,34,64] may not cause a beneficial increase in parasympathetic-mediated tone as assessed by heart rate variability.[65] This suggests that ACE inhibitors might have a greater effect on arrhythmias, at least compared with modest doses of ARBs.

Uricosuric effect

The apparently specific uricosuric effect of losartan[66,67] could do more than just protect against gout. Plasma concentrations of uric acid may be a marker of oxidant stress[68] that in turn may have adverse effects on cardiac and vascular function. Whether these properties are shared by other ARBs is not clear as yet.

Tolerability

ARBs may be better tolerated than, at least, some ACE inhibitors.[69] Only if a drug is taken can it be effective and therefore greater tolerability may translate into greater efficacy. ARBs have generally been better tolerated than placebo in studies of hypertension, although it should be pointed out that less patients have generally been withdrawn from ACE inhibitors than placebo in studies of CHF.

Will the combination of ACE inhibitors and ARBs prove superior to either class used alone?

Renin secretion is suppressed by stimulation of AII receptor, and AT_1 receptor antagonists increase plasma renin by releasing it from this negative feedback loop. As renin rises, so does angiotensin I, and, consequently, AII.[69,70] Just as the effects of ACE inhibition may be overcome by competition from rising concentrations of angiotensin I, so AT_1 inhibition may be overcome by rising concentrations of AII, either by displacing ARBs that bind reversibly to the AT_1 receptor or by stimulating unblocked receptors more powerfully. Also, it is possible that excessive stimulation of unblocked AT_2 receptors could be harmful.

Rather than being alternatives it is possible that the actions of ARBs and ACE inhibitors are complementary. ACE inhibition could attenuate the rise in AII associated with ARBs, thereby reducing competition for binding of the ARB to the AT_1 receptor and protecting unblocked AT_1 receptors, whereas ARBs could block the effects of any residual AII formed despite ACE inhibition. Studies show that the rise in AII induced by an ARB can be attenuated by ACE inhibition, at least in the short term, while addition of an ARB to an ACE inhibitor results in a further decline in aldosterone, indicating better renin–angiotensin system blockade.[3,71]

The question of dose

Surprisingly, after 15 years of research we still know comparatively little about the optimal dose of any ACE inhibitor for CHF.[72–74] This is a very important issue because, when comparing the effects of two classes of drugs, it is important to know that merely changing the dose of one or other drug would not have replicated any difference observed or if no difference was observed that this did not reflect the use of an inadequate dose of one or other drug. The NETWORK study showed no difference in outcome from 2.5 mg, 5 mg, or 10 mg twice daily of enalapril over 6 months, whereas the ATLAS study suggested a greater morbidity/mortality benefit with 35 mg compared with 5 mg/day of lisinopril over 46 months.[72,73] However, these studies still do not show what is the optimal long-term dose of an ACE inhibitor.

Landmark trials and meta-analyses principally designed to compare ARBs with placebo in the absence of an ACE inhibitor (Tables 9.1, 9.2a, and 9.2b; Figures 9.2–9.5)

This section includes two landmark trials addressing this question, CHARM-alternative[6] and CHARM-preserved,[7,10] and two meta-analyses of smaller trials, one of losartan[23] and the other of candesartan.[24] The VAL-HeFT study included a subgroup of patients who were not taking ACE inhibitors.[75] This study is dealt with in the section focusing on ARBs added to ACE inhibitors. Apart from the CHARM-preserved trial, comparing candesartan and placebo in patients with heart failure and preserved left ventricular systolic function, these trials all focused on heart failure due to left ventricular systolic dysfunction (LVSD). The I-PRESERVE trial[76] is also investigating the effects of an ARB, irbesartan, in patients with heart failure and preserved left ventricular systolic function and, as in CHARM-preserved, some use of ACE inhibitors is allowed. It is unlikely to report for some years.

The losartan meta-analysis[23]

This meta-analysis consisted of six randomized, double-blind trials in patients with heart failure due to LVSD, three of which compared losartan (mostly 50 mg/day) with placebo and comprised 890 patients with 12 weeks of follow-up. One was a dose-ranging hemodynamic study and the others had exercise capacity as their primary end point. About half of patients had previously received an ACE inhibitor, but this treatment had been discontinued either because of side effects or in order for the patient to qualify for study entry. These trials were conducted prior to widespread use of β-blockers. The mean age of the patients was 62 years, about 70% were men, and coronary disease was the predominant etiology of their LVSD. The meta-analysis showed a significant reduction in mortality with losartan compared with placebo (1.8% vs 4.7%; $p = 0.014$).

The hemodynamic study showed that after 3 months therapy and 12 hours following a further dose, 25 mg of losartan reduced systemic vascular resistance by about 20%, pulmonary capillary wedge pressure (PCWP) by 5 mmHg, blood pressure by 6 mmHg, and heart rate by 6 bpm (all placebo-corrected), and increased cardiac index by about 0.4 L/min/m.[70] The 50 mg dose exerted similar, but no greater an effect. Other doses exerted less consistent effects. Only the 50 mg dose reduced cardiothoracic ratio significantly over 3 months. Thus, as with ACE inhibitors, the long-term hemodynamic benefits were generally modest. Reductions in aldosterone were observed after 12 weeks of the 10 mg, 25 mg, and 50 mg doses of losartan. Increases in renin and angiotensin II that appeared after acute dosing were not present after 12 weeks. Norepinephrine changed little if at all. The 25 mg and 50 mg doses of losartan reduced plasma concentrations of N-terminal pro-atrial natriuretic peptide, and this correlated with the decline in PCWP.[77]

The hemodynamic study but not the exercise testing studies showed an improvement in symptoms. Neither exercise testing study showed an improvement in exercise capacity, but it is

Table 9.1
Study design of and baseline characteristics of patients included in landmark trials of heart failure comparing ARB with placebo in the absence (mainly) of an ACE inhibitor.

	CHARM-alternative[6,7]	Val-HeFT (subgroup)[75]	CHARM-preserved[7,10]
Comparison	Candesartan vs placebo	Valsartan vs placebo	Candesartan vs placebo
n	2028	366	3023
Follow-up (months)	33.7	23	36.6
Mean age (years)	67	67	67
≥75 years old (%)	23	63*	27
Women (%)	32	29	40
NYHA (II/III/IV shown as %)	47/49/4	53/47[†]	61/37/2
Mean LVEF (entry criterion in brackets)	30 (≤40%)	28 (<40%)	54 (>40%)
Mean systolic blood pressure (mmHg)	130	126	136
Main cause of heart failure			
Ischemic heart disease	68	68	56
Idiopathic	20	–	9
Hypertension	6	–	23
Other	6	–	2
Medical history			
Diabetes	27	–	28
Atrial fibrillation	25	–	29
Hypertension	50	–	64
Current angina	23	–	28
Pacemaker	9	–	7
Implantable defibrillator	3	–	1
CABG	25	–	22
Treatment			
Diuretic	85	–	75
ACE inhibitors	Excluded	Excluded	19
Beta-blockers	55	38	56
Spironolactone	24	–	12
Calcium channel blocker	16	–	31
Digoxin	46	–	28
Anticoagulant	31	–	25
Aspirin	58	–	58
Statin	42	–	42

*≥65 years rather than ≥75 years.
[†]Data for NYHA III/IV combined.
–, Data not reported.

Table 9.2a
Summary of outcome of landmark trials of heart failure (HF) comparing ARB with placebo in the absence of an ACE inhibitor in patients with left ventricular systolic dysfunction.

	Patients		Follow-up (months)	Mortality		Total no. of hospitalizations		Death or HF hospitalization: no. (%) of patients		Total HF hospitalizations	
	Placebo	ARB		Placebo	ARB	Placebo	ARB	Placebo	ARB	Placebo	ARB
Losartan meta-analysis[23]	274	616	3	13 (4.7%)	11 (1.8%)	–	–	–	–	–	–
Candesartan meta-analysis[24]	606	1287	3	11 (1.8%)	20 (1.6%)	–	–	43 (7.1%)	56 (4.4%)	–	–
Val-HeFT subset[75]	181	185	23	49 (27.1%)	32 (17.3%)	262	199	77 (42.5%)	46 (24.9%)	117	51
CHARM-alternative[6]	1015	1013	34	296 (29.2%)	265 (26.2%)	1835	1718	433 (42.7%)	371 (36.6%)	608	445
Japanese candesartan study[80]	144	148	5	3 (2.1%)	2 (1.4%)	–	–	13 (9.0%)	31 (20.9%)	–	–
Total	**2220**	**3249**		**372 (16.8%)**	**330 (10.2%)**	**2097**	**1917**	**566 (29.1%)**	**504 (19.1%)**	**725**	**496**

Table 9.2b
Summary of outcome of landmark trials of heart failure (HF) comparing ARB with placebo in patients with preserved left ventricular systolic dysfunction.

	Patients		Follow-up (months)	Mortality		Total no. of hospitalizations		Death or HF hospitalization: no. (%) of patients		Total HF hospitalizations	
	Placebo	ARB		Placebo	ARB	Placebo	ARB	Placebo	ARB	Placebo	ARB
CHARM-Preserved[10]	1509	1514	36	237 (15.7%)	244 (16.1%)	2545	2510	366 (24.3%)	333 (22.0%)	566	402

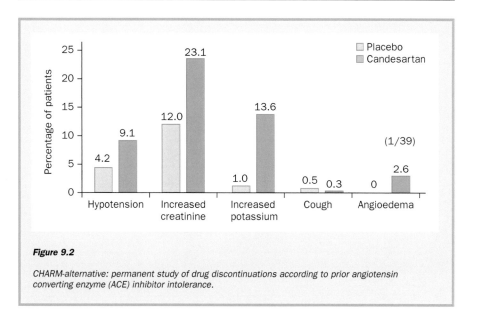

Figure 9.2

CHARM-alternative: permanent study of drug discontinuations according to prior angiotensin converting enzyme (ACE) inhibitor intolerance.

difficult to show improvement in exercise capacity with treatment in patients who have few symptoms or only minor exercise limitation. It is possible that patients with more severe symptoms were not enrolled by investigators due to concerns about placing them on placebo for 3 months.

In summary, these trials suggested that losartan might improve morbidity and mortality and possibly symptoms in patients with heart failure when used instead of an ACE inhibitor. Although the hemodynamic study suggested that 50 mg/day of losartan was at the top of the dose response, fewer than 30 patients were studied at each dose.

The candesartan meta-analysis[24]

This meta-analysis consisted of five randomized, double-blind trials (including STRETCH[78] and SPICE[79]) in patients with heart failure due to LVSD. Four trials, comprising 1189 patients, compared candesartan in doses ranging from 2 to 16 mg/day against placebo without background ACE inhibitor. The mean age of the patients was 63 years old, and most were men with coronary disease and predominantly mild symptoms. The largest trial (STRETCH; $n = 844$), lasted 12 weeks and the longest trial, 52 weeks ($n = 463$). Two trials included only ACE inhibitor-intolerant patients.

The meta-analysis showed no effect of candesartan on mortality, which was low overall (1.8% on placebo vs 1.6% on candesartan). All-cause hospitalization was also unaffected but

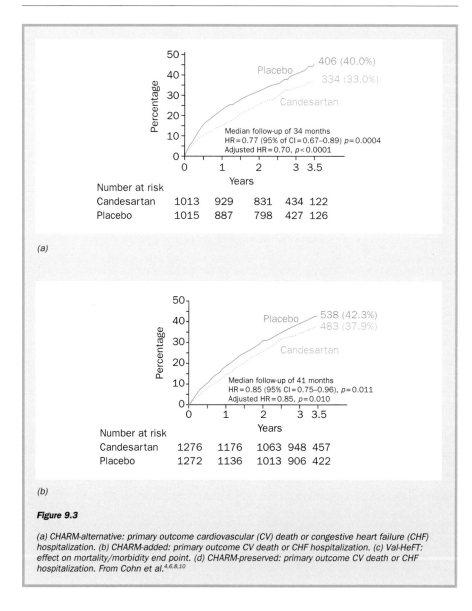

Figure 9.3

(a) CHARM-alternative: primary outcome cardiovascular (CV) death or congestive heart failure (CHF) hospitalization. (b) CHARM-added: primary outcome CV death or CHF hospitalization. (c) Val-HeFT: effect on mortality/morbidity end point. (d) CHARM-preserved: primary outcome CV death or CHF hospitalization. From Cohn et al.[4,6,8,10]

candesartan appeared effective in reducing the number of patients requiring hospitalization for acute decompensation of heart failure (3.5% vs 1.1%; $p = 0.002$).

Compared to placebo, candesartan improved symptoms and exercise capacity in the STRETCH study,[78] with the highest dose (16 mg/day) having the greatest effect. Adverse effects were no more common even with the highest dose of candesartan compared with placebo and only two patients required treatment to be withdrawn for an adverse effect.

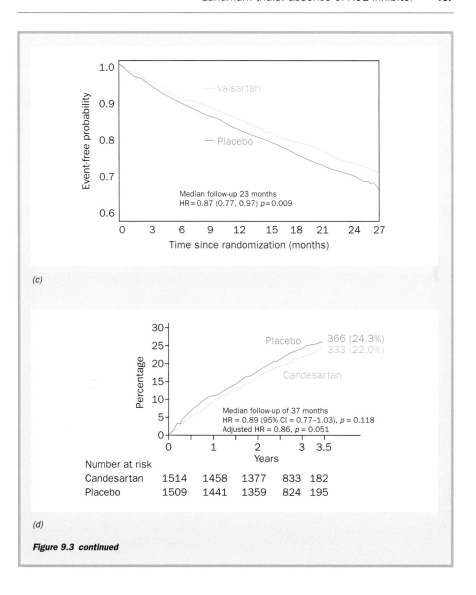

(c)

(d)

Figure 9.3 continued

The SPICE study[79] screened 9580 patients with CHF and ejection fraction ≤35% to identify ACE-intolerant patients: 9% of patients were found to be intolerant of ACE inhibitors, mainly due to cough or hypotension; 179 patients were randomized to candesartan (titrated to 16 mg/day) or placebo and followed for 12–14 weeks. No effect on symptoms, morbidity, or mortality were observed but the study was inadequately powered to do so.

Detailed reports on the other component studies have not been published. A subsequent long-term study, not included in this meta-analysis,[80–82] compared placebo and candesartan

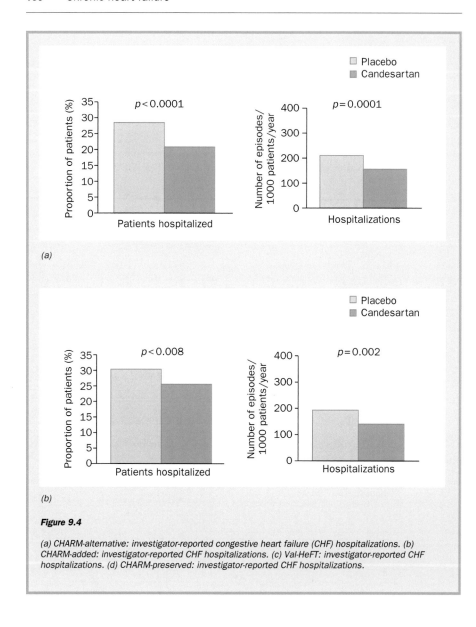

Figure 9.4

(a) CHARM-alternative: investigator-reported congestive heart failure (CHF) hospitalizations. (b) CHARM-added: investigator-reported CHF hospitalizations. (c) Val-HeFT: investigator-reported CHF hospitalizations. (d) CHARM-preserved: investigator-reported CHF hospitalizations.

(8 mg/day) in 305 Japanese patients with predominantly mild heart failure. Candesartan was associated with a reduction in worsening heart failure.

In summary, these trials suggested that candesartan might improve symptoms and possibly morbidity in patients with heart failure when used instead of an ACE inhibitor. The low event rate precludes any comment on mortality.

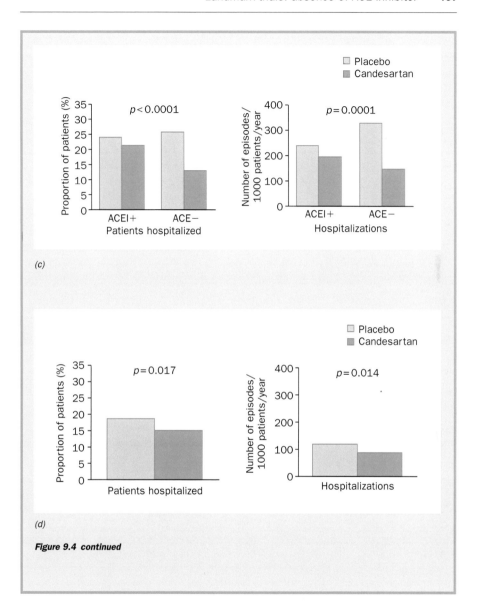

(c)

(d)

Figure 9.4 continued

CHARM-alternative[6,7]

The CHARM program consisted of three separate randomized, double-blind clinical trials that were also designed to be analyzed as a single outcome trial.[9,83] However, as each component study asks a different, clinically relevant question, the trials are probably best interpreted individually rather than as a whole. Also, all-cause mortality, the primary end point of the

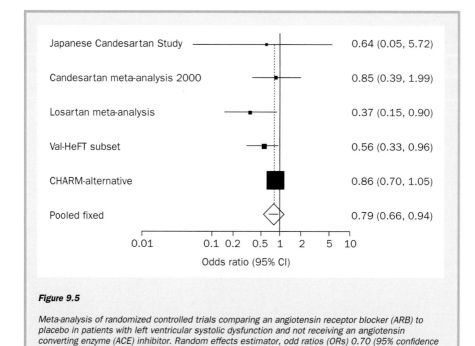

Figure 9.5

Meta-analysis of randomized controlled trials comparing an angiotensin receptor blocker (ARB) to placebo in patients with left ventricular systolic dysfunction and not receiving an angiotensin converting enzyme (ACE) inhibitor. Random effects estimator, odd ratios (ORs) 0.70 (95% confidence interval (CIs) = 0.43 to 1.00).

overall analysis,[9] was not reduced significantly by candesartan using the principal pre-planned analysis, which was not adjusted for covariates.

CHARM-alternative included patients with symptomatic heart failure due to LVSD who had a history of ACE inhibitor intolerance, predominantly ACE inhibitor-induced cough (72%). Candesartan was initiated at 4 mg/day (81% of patients) or 8 mg/day, according to the discretion of the investigator, and then titrated at not more than 2-week intervals to 32 mg/day. Measurement of serum potassium and creatinine was recommended during titration. Patients were monitored long-term at 4-monthly intervals. The primary end point was cardiovascular death or unplanned admission to hospital for the management of worsening heart failure. This was defined as admission with documented worsening symptoms or signs and requiring treatment with intravenous diuretics.

A total of 2028 patients were randomized and followed for a mean of 33.7 months. Only 3 patients were lost to follow-up. The mean age of the patients was 67 years old and 23% were aged ≥75 years old. Most patients were men and had coronary disease. Of those randomized to candesartan, 55% were taking a β-blocker (rising to 64% during the course of the study) and 25% were taking spironolactone (unchanged during the study on candesartan but increasing to 29% on placebo); 59% of patients randomized to candesartan vs 73% randomized to placebo were on the target dose at 6 months. Adverse events led to withdrawal of study medication in 22% and 19% of patients randomized to candesartan and placebo, respectively. However, patients who had previously withdrawn from ACE inhibitors because of cough or angioedema rarely discontinued study medication because of adverse events. In each group, 6% of patients started an open-label ACE inhibitor and 9% an open-label ARB. Patients randomized to candesartan were more likely to withdraw for hypotension (3.7% vs 0.9%), renal dysfunction (6.1% vs 2.7%), and hyperkalemia (1.9% vs 0.3%), and these events were most likely to occur in patients who had previously discontinued ACE inhibitors for these problems (see Figure 9.2). Serum creatinine more than doubled in 5.5% of patients (vs 1.6% on placebo) and serum potassium increased to $\geq$6 mmol/L in 3% of patients (vs 1.3% on placebo). Candesartan reduced systolic blood pressure by a mean of 4 mmHg.

The absolute risk reduction (ARR) in the primary end point with candesartan was 7.0% or a relative risk reduction (RRR) of 23% ($p = 0.004$), increasing to 30% after adjusting for imbalances between randomized groups in patients' baseline characteristics (see Figure 9.3 and Table 9.2a). This effect was brought about by a somewhat greater effect on heart failure hospitalizations (ARR = 7.8%; RRR = 39%; $p < 0.0001$ adjusted for covariates) and a slightly lesser effect on cardiovascular death (ARR = 3.2%; RRR = 20%; $p = 0.02$ adjusted). The total number of investigator-defined hospital admissions for heart failure was reduced by 56 events (from 211 to 155) per 1000 patients per year ($p = 0.0001$) (see Figure 9.4), which is very similar to the effect of enalapril compared with placebo in SOLVD treatment (reduced by 65 events from 219 to 154 events per 1000 patients per year).[84]

Candesartan was associated with slightly more myocardial infarctions ($n = 75$ vs 48; $p = 0.025$) but not strokes ($n = 36$ vs 42), although few patients suffered either event. This might suggest that candesartan, unlike ACE inhibitors,[39,85,86] does not reduce vascular events in this setting but as candesartan was associated with somewhat fewer cardiovascular deaths these data need to be interpreted with caution.

All-cause mortality was reduced, although this was significant only after adjusting for covariates (ARR = 3.1%; RRR = 17% adjusted; $p = 0.033$). The predominant effect on mode of death was a reduction in sudden death, with a smaller benefit from reducing worsening heart failure.[12] There was a trend to more deaths due to myocardial infarction and no difference in the rate of cancer deaths (<1% per year). The reduction in heart failure admissions was reflected in a strong trend for a reduction in all-cause hospitalization ($p = 0.06$). Secondary analysis indicate an improvement in symptoms with, on average, 1 in every 14 patients reporting a substantial improvement in symptoms. Gains seemed greater in women, older patients, those with initially milder symptoms, and amongst patients not taking β-blockers, although subgroup analysis was not significant.

In summary, this trial suggests that candesartan at doses of 16 × 32 mg/day is reasonably well tolerated, substantially more effective than placebo, and, at these doses, as effective as an ACE inhibitor would have been had it been tolerated.[81,82] Caution is required in extrapolating these results to patients who have been withdrawn from ACE inhibitors because of hypotension or renal dysfunction or in extrapolating these data to infer that ARBs may be used in preference to an ACE inhibitor in a patient who does not exhibit ACE inhibitor intolerance. As the trial was analyzed on an intention-to-treat basis and a substantial number of patients randomized to placebo subsequently received treatment with an ACE inhibitor or ARB, the trial underestimates the true magnitude of benefit that should be observed in clinical practice.

Overall, this group of trials suggest that, compared with placebo, ARBs improve symptoms, reduce hospitalizations (see Figure 9.4), and lower mortality (see Figure 9.5).[81,82]

CHARM-preserved[7,10]

This is the first substantial trial to assess the effects of treatment in patients with a clinical syndrome suggestive of heart failure but in whom heart failure due to LVSD or major valve disease has been excluded. Epidemiologic studies suggest that up to half of patients with heart failure belong to this category and predict that this group should be older and predominantly female.[87] Follow-up studies have suggested that this group of patients have a better short-term survival but that longer-term survival may be as poor as for patients with LVSD and that they have a high rate of hospitalization for heart failure.[76,88] CHARM-preserved is therefore of special scientific interest. However, it is likely that the patients enrolled in this study are a highly heterogeneous group of patients, including many with a misdiagnosis of heart failure, patients with forme fruste systolic dysfunction, and perhaps some patients with isolated diastolic dysfunction.[76]

CHARM-preserved included patients with symptomatic heart failure who had been hospitalized at some time in the past for a cardiac problem (69% had a previous admission with heart failure) and who had a left ventricular ejection fraction (LVEF) >40%. Candesartan was initiated at 4 mg/day (75% of patients) or 8 mg/day, according to the discretion of the investigator, and then titrated at not more than 2-week intervals to 32 mg/day. Measurement of serum potassium and creatinine was recommended during titration. Patients were monitored long term at 4-monthly intervals. The primary end point was cardiovascular (CV) death or unplanned admission to hospital for the management of worsening heart failure, as defined above.

A total of 3205 patients were randomized and followed for a mean of 36.6 months. Only 3 patients were lost to follow-up. The mean age of the patients was 67 years old and 27% were aged ≥75 years old; 60% of the patients were men and 44% had experienced a myocardial infarction. Of those randomized to candesartan, 56% were taking a β-blocker at baseline (falling to 47% during the course of the study) and 11% were taking spironolactone (falling to 9% during the course of the study). Also, 19% of patients were taking an ACE inhibitor at baseline, which rose to around 24% during the study in both groups. In each group, 3% of patients started an open-label ARB: 67% of patients randomized to candesartan vs 79% randomized to placebo were on the target dose at 6 months; 18% of those randomized to candesartan vs 14% of those randomized to placebo discontinued trial medication because of an adverse event. Patients randomized to candesartan were more likely to withdraw for hypotension (2.4% vs 1.1%), renal dysfunction (4.8% vs 2.4%), and hyperkalemia (1.5% vs 0.6%). Serum creatinine more than doubled in 6% of patients (vs 3% on placebo) and serum potassium increased to ≥ 6 mmol/L in 2% of patients (vs 1% on placebo). Candesartan reduced systolic blood pressure by a mean of 7 mmHg.

The annual event rate for the primary end point in the placebo group was 9.1%, half that observed in CHARM-alternative (see Figure 9.3). The absolute reduction in the primary end point with candesartan was just 2.0% or a relative reduction of 11% (NS), increasing to 14% ($p = 0.051$) after adjusting for imbalances between randomized groups in patients' baseline characteristics. There was no effect on mortality, but a trend for an effect on heart failure hospitalizations (ARR = 2.4%; RRR = 16% adjusted; $p = 0.047$) (see Table 9.2b). Sudden death accounted for slightly more deaths than worsening heart failure.[12] The total number of investigator-defined hospital admissions for heart failure was reduced by 36 (123 vs 87) events per 1000 patients per year ($p = 0.014$) (see Figure 9.4). No effect of candesartan on vascular events such as myocardial infraction or stroke was observed. All-cause mortality and all-cause hospitalization were both unchanged by candesartan. The non-cardiovascular death rate was similar to that observed in the other component trials of the CHARM program, but the cardiovascular mortality was half that observed in trials of LVSD.[12] The proportion of hospitalizations that was non-cardiovascular was also substantially greater in this study than in the CHARM-alternative. There was also little evidence that candesartan improved symptoms. Fewer patients developed diabetes on candesartan in the overall trial, and this was predominantly due to a reduction in this patient group.[11]

In summary, this trial suggests that candesartan may have some modest effect on altering the natural history of heart failure with preserved left ventricular systolic function. It is possible that stricter entry criteria that required more substantial evidence of cardiac dysfunction would have identified patients with greater benefit. An analysis of the data including only patients who were not receiving an ACE inhibitor would also be valuable.

I-PRESERVE

This is a randomized, double-blind study comparing irbesartan (target dose 300 mg/day) with placebo in patients with heart failure but without LVSD. It is similar, in terms of design, patients recruited, and intention, to CHARM-preserved. It is unlikely to report for some years. It is difficult to see why the outcome of this trial would be substantially different to CHARM-preserved, although the size and the duration of the trial could make a difference to the confidence intervals (CIs) around the effect.

Landmark trials principally designed to compare ARBs with placebo in the presence of an ACE inhibitor (Tables 9.3 and 9.4; Figures 9.3–9.7)

The Val-HeFT[4,5,75,89–93] and CHARM-added[7,8] trials are included here. The RESOLVD[3,82] and VALIANT studies[27,28] have complex designs, including a comparison of combined ACE inhibitor/ARB against each agent used alone, and these trials will also be discussed.

RESOLVD[3,28]

RESOLVD was a complex randomized, double-blind, dose-ranging study that compared enalapril 10 mg twice daily to three doses of candesartan (4 mg, 8 mg, and 16 mg/day) in the absence of an ACE inhibitor and two doses of candesartan (4 mg and 8 mg/day) in addition to enalapril 10 mg twice daily. The comparison of the combination with either agent used alone is the focus of this section. The starting dose of candesartan was 2 mg/day and of enalapril 2.5 mg twice daily. Patients with symptomatic heart failure and an LVEF <40% were eligible. The 'primary' end points included exercise distance (6-minute corridor walk), cardiac function, neuroendocrine measures, symptoms, and quality of life. Morbidity and mortality were safety outcomes. After 17 weeks, patients not taking β-blockers were eligible for re-randomization to placebo or metoprolol in addition to their initial study medication.[3]

A total of 436 patients were randomized to either enalapril or candesartan alone and a further 332 to the combination. Patients were followed for 43 weeks overall. Patients were predominantly men and most had few symptoms (63% in NYHA class II). More than 90% of patients had been withdrawn from ACE inhibitors to enter the study.

Compared to either candesartan or enalapril used alone, the combination did not improve exercise distance, LVEF, norepinephrine, endothelin, symptoms, or quality of life. The latter may reflect the mild severity of symptoms at baseline. However, compared with either agent alone, the combination did inhibit progressive ventricular dilation and this was associated with a greater and more sustained reduction in brain natriuretic peptide, with similar trends for aldosterone. The highest dose of candesartan exerted the greatest effect. These effects were associated with about a 5 mmHg greater reduction in systolic blood pressure.

RESOLVD was stopped prematurely due to a higher incidence of death in the candesartan (6.1%) and combination groups (8.7%) than in the enalapril group (3.7%), although no similar trend was noted for hospitalization.

In summary, the mechanistic data from this study suggested that combination therapy might be superior to either agent used alone. The excess mortality with combination therapy, in hindsight, most probably reflects a spuriously low mortality in the small number ($n = 107$) of

Table 9.3
Study design of and baseline characteristics of patients included in landmark trials of heart failure comparing ARB with placebo in addition to an ACE inhibitor.

	Val-HeFT (Main)[4]	CHARM-alternative[7,8]	RESOLVD[3] *
Comparison	Valsartan vs placebo	Candesartan vs placebo	Candesartan vs placebo
n	5010	2548	441
Mean follow-up (months)	23	41	10
Mean age (years)	63	64	63
≥75 years old (%)	–	18	–
Women (%)	20	21	13
NYHA (II/III/IV shown as %)	62/36/2	24/73/3	63/35/2
Mean LVEF (entry criterion in brackets)	27 (<40%)	28 (≤40%)	28 (<40%)
Mean systolic blood pressure (mmHg)	124	125	120
Cause of heart failure			
Ischemic heart disease	57	62	72
Idiopathic	31	26	17
Hypertension	7	7	–
Other	5	5	11
Medical history			
Diabetes	26	30	–
Atrial fibrillation	12	27	–
Hypertension	–	48	–
Current angina	–	20	–
Pacemaker	–	9	–
Implantable defibrillator	–	4	–
CABG	–	25	–
Treatment			
Diuretic	86	90	85
ACE inhibitors	93	100	Excluded at baseline
Beta-blockers	35	55	13% on combination vs 23% on enalapril ($p < 0.05$)
Spironolactone	–	17	–
Calcium channel blocker	–	10	15
Digoxin	67	58	69
Anticoagulant	–	38	31
Aspirin	–	51	53
Statin	–	41	–

*Includes only patients randomized to combination or enalapril.

Table 9.4
Summary of outcome of landmark trials of heart failure comparing ARB with placebo or control when added to an ACE inhibitor.

	Patients		Follow-up (months)	Mortality		Total no. of hospitalizations		Death or HF hospitalization: no. (%) of patients		Total HF hospitalizations	
	Placebo	ARB		Placebo	ARB	Placebo	ARB	Placebo	ARB	Placebo	ARB
RESOLVD[3]	109	332	11	4 (3.7%)	29 (8.7%)	–	–	10 (9.2%)	58 (17.5%)	–	–
Val-HeFT-main*[4]	2318	2326	23	435 (18.8%)	463 (19.9%)	2844	2657	724 (31.2%)	677 (29.1%)	1072	872
CHARM-added[8]	1272	1276	41	412 (32.4%)	377 (29.5%)	2798	2462	587 (46.1%)	539 (42.2%)	836	607
Total for heart failure	**3699**	**3934**		**851 (23.0%)**	**869 (22.1%)**	**5642**	**5119**	**1321 (35.7%)**	**1274 (32.4%)**	**1908**	**1479**
VALIANT[4,27]	4909	4885	25	958 (19.5%)	941 (19.3%)	–	–	1335 (27.2%)	1331 (27.2%)	–	–
Overall total	**8608**	**8819**		**1809 (21.0%)**	**1810 (20.5%)**	**5642**	**5119**	**2656 (30.9%)**	**2605 (29.5%)**	**1908**	**1479**

*Patients not on ACE inhibitors have been excluded.

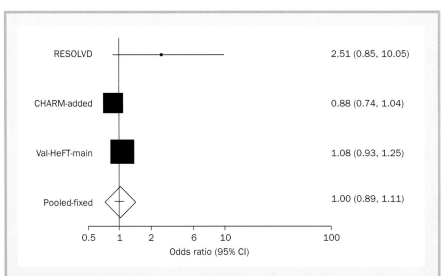

Figure 9.6

Angiotensin receptor blocker (ARB) with background angiotensin converting enzyme (ACE) inhibitor in patients with left ventricular systolic dysfunction. Analysis of ARB vs control with background ACE inhibitor. Odd ratios (ORs) and 95% confidence intervals (CIs).
Only patients who were not taking an ACE inhibitor in the Val-HeFT-main study are included in this analysis. Full random effects estimator is 1.08 (95% CI 0.62–2.60). Some evidence of heterogeneity (p for heterogeneity = 0.0405).

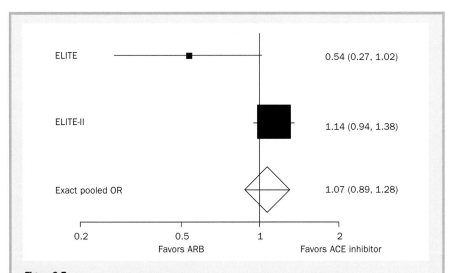

Figure 9.7

Angiotensin receptor blocker (ARB) vs angiotensin converting enzyme (ACE) in trials of chronic heart failure. Odd ratios (OR) and 95% confidence intervals (CIs). Evidence of heterogeneity between included trials made interpretation of the meta-analysis questionable.

patients randomized to enalapril alone and a somewhat higher than expected mortality in the group randomized to enalapril in combination with 8 mg/day of candesartan. At the time, it caused considerable concern.

Val-HeFT [4,5,75,89–93]

The Val-HeFT study compared valsartan (target dose 160 mg twice daily) with placebo, predominantly in patients who were taking substantial doses (e.g. a mean of 17 mg/day of enalapril) of ACE inhibitors (93%) in patients with treated symptomatic heart failure due to LVSD; 7% of patients were not taking an ACE inhibitor at baseline, presumably mainly because of previous intolerance.

Valsartan was initiated at 40 mg twice daily and then titrated at 2-week intervals to a target of 160 mg twice daily provided the patient had no hypotensive symptoms, the standing systolic blood pressure was >90 mmHg, and renal function had not deteriorated substantially (e.g. 50% increase in creatinine). Patients were monitored long term at 3-monthly intervals. The co-primary end points were all-cause mortality and the composite of death, hospitalization for heart failure, resuscitated cardiac arrest, or the administration of intravenous inotropic or vasodilator agents for more than 4 hours without hospitalization. The latter two components of the composite contributed little to the outcome.

A total of 5010 patients were randomized and followed for a mean of 23 months. The mean age of the patients was 63 years old and 47% were aged >65 years old. Most patients were men and had coronary disease. Of those randomized to valsartan, 35% were taking a β-blocker and only 5% were taking spironolactone; 84% of patients randomized to valsartan vs 93% of those randomized to placebo achieved the target dose. Adverse events led to withdrawal of study medication in 9.9% and 7.2% of patients randomized to valsartan and placebo, respectively. Patients randomized to valsartan were more likely to withdraw for hypotension (1.3% vs 0.8%) and renal dysfunction (1.1% vs 0.2%). Serum creatinine and serum potassium increased by an average of only 7 μmol/L and 0.05 mmol/L, respectively, compared with placebo. Valsartan reduced systolic blood pressure by a mean of 4 mmHg compared with placebo at 4 months and 1 year.

Valsartan had no overall effect on mortality but a statistically significant reduction ($p = 0.017$) (on a log-rank test) was noted in the small subgroup of patients who were not taking an ACE inhibitor at baseline[75] (see Table 9.2a). There was no effect on mortality in patients taking ACE inhibitors at baseline in the absence of a β-blocker and an excess mortality when added to both an ACE inhibitor and β-blocker.[4,5,19]

Valsartan reduced the composite morbidity/mortality outcome (ARR = 4.4%; RRR = 13%; $p = 0.009$) almost entirely due to a reduction in hospitalization with heart failure (RRR = 24%;

$p = 0.001$) (see Figure 9.3). The total number of investigator-defined hospital admissions for heart failure was reduced by 55 (from 241 to 196) events per 1000 patients per year ($p = 0.002$) (Figure 9.4). A greater effect was observed in patients not taking ACE inhibitors and in patients taking lower doses of ACE inhibitors with little evidence of an effect in patients on full doses of ACE inhibitors.[19] Non heart failure admissions were unaffected, but this was enough to dilute the effect on heart failure admissions so that the trend to a reduction in all-cause hospitalization was not significant.[90]

Patients taking a combination of β-blockers and ACE inhibitors at baseline had a higher mortality if randomized to valsartan. However, it is likely that many patients had β-blockers initiated during the study and so interaction with baseline therapy should be interpreted with care. In the light of subsequent data, it is almost certain that this was a chance finding. Other subgroup analyses revealed no significant heterogeneity in the effect of valsartan. Patients with higher NYHA class, lower LVEF, and more dilated left ventricles tended to have more benefit, perhaps reflecting the fact that they were sicker and had more cardiovascular events to prevent. Patients with ischemic heart disease and those with diabetes tended to have less benefit, perhaps suggesting that ARBs have a limited effect on vascular protection or an adverse effect of excessive blood pressure reduction in patients with severe coronary disease.

Valsartan improved symptoms using a variety of measures and quality of life.[20] The effect on symptoms was equivalent to improving 1 in every 20 patients by one full NYHA class ($p < 0.001$), which is probably a worthwhile benefit (see Figure 9.6). Progressive increases in plasma concentrations of brain natriuretic peptide (BNP) and norepinephrine, markers of a worse prognosis, were noted on placebo.[89,91] Valsartan produced a sustained reduction in BNP and attenuated the increase in norepinephrine.[19] These effects were most prominent in patients who were not taking ACE inhibitors, but were also observed in the presence of ACE inhibitors and β-blockers. Most patients in the study had serial echocardiographic measurements of left ventricular function. These showed that valsartan increased LVEF by about 1.3% (placebo subtracted: i.e. from about 26.6% to 31.1% on valsartan compared with 26.9% to 30.1% on placebo) ($p < 0.0001$).[4,92] Again, effects were greatest in the absence of an ACE inhibitor and absent in patients taking both a β-blocker and an ACE inhibitor. Similarly, valsartan reduced left ventricular diastolic dimension by $7 \, mm/m^2$, with the effect being greatest in those not taking ACE inhibitors and least in those taking ACE inhibitors and β-blockers.[92] Clinical and functional benefits appeared similar in younger and older patients.[18] Improvement of cardiac function also reduced the risk of developing atrial fibrillation, an adverse prognostic sign in patients with heart failure.[21]

In summary, although this trial shows that valsartan at a dose of 160 mg twice daily is well tolerated, safe, improves symptoms, and reduces hospitalization for heart failure when added to an ACE inhibitor, it raises concerns about triple therapy in combination with β-blockers.

CHARM-added[7,8]

The CHARM-added study compared candesartan (target dose 32 mg/day) with placebo in patients who were taking substantial doses (e.g. a mean of 17 mg/day of enalapril) of ACE inhibitors in patients with symptomatic heart failure due to LVSD. To exclude patients at a low risk of events, patients who were in NYHA class II had to have had an admission for a cardiac problem in the previous 6 months.

Candesartan was initiated at 4 mg/day (86% of patients) or 8 mg/day, according to the discretion of the investigator, and then titrated at not more than 2-week intervals to 32 mg/day. Measurement of serum potassium and creatinine was recommended during titration. Patients were monitored long term at 4-monthly intervals. The primary end point was CV death or unplanned admission to hospital for the management of worsening heart failure, as defined above.

A total of 2548 patients were randomized and followed for a mean of 41 months. Only 4 patients were lost to follow-up. The mean age of the patients was 64 years and 18% were aged >75 years. Most patients were men and had coronary disease. Of those randomized to candesartan, 55% were taking a β-blocker (rising to 64% during the course of the study) and 17% were taking spironolactone (rising to 20% on candesartan and 25% on placebo); 61% of patients randomized to candesartan vs 73% randomized to placebo were on the target dose at 6 months. Adverse events led to withdrawal of study medication in 24% and 18% of patients randomized to candesartan and placebo, respectively. In each group, 6% of patients started an open-label ACE inhibitor and 9% an open-label ARB. Patients randomized to candesartan were more likely to withdraw for hypotension (4.5% vs 3.1%), renal dysfunction (7.8% vs 4.1%), and hyperkalemia (3.4% vs 0.7%). Serum creatinine more than doubled in 7% of patients (vs 6% on placebo) and serum potassium increased to $\geq$6 mmol/L in 3% of patients (vs 1% on placebo). These effects were not substantially different in the presence of spironolactone. Candesartan reduced systolic blood pressure by a mean of 5 mmHg by 6 months, with no greater effect observed in those patients taking β-blockers.

The absolute reduction in the primary end point with candesartan was 4.4% or a relative reduction of 15% ($p = 0.011$) (see Figure 9.3). This effect was brought about by very similar effects on heart failure hospitalizations and CV death. Benefits tended to be greater in patients receiving β-blockers and higher doses of ACE inhibitors. The total number of investigator-defined hospital admissions for heart failure was reduced by 53 (from 192 to 139) events per 1000 patients per year ($p = 0.002$) (see Figure 9.4). Candesartan was associated with slightly fewer myocardial infarctions ($n = 44$ vs 69; $p = 0.012$) but not strokes ($n = 47$ vs 41), although few patients suffered either event. The total number of admissions was reduced ($p = 0.023$). A trend to a reduction in all-cause mortality was not significant. The trend was identical in the presence or absence of a β-blocker. Sudden death was the most common mode of death.[12]

Addition of candesartan improved symptoms[13,14] and, on average, about 1 patient in every 12 appeared to get substantial benefit.

In summary, this trial suggests that candesartan at a target dose of 32 mg/day is well tolerated, safe, improves symptoms, and reduces hospitalizations when added to ACE inhibitors with or without β-blockers. This trial provides no definitive evidence of a mortality benefit with ARBs in this clinical setting.

VALIANT[27,28,81] (see Tables 9.4, 9.6, and 9.7[4,27,28])

This trial compared valsartan (160 mg twice daily) with captopril (50 mg three times a day) and the combination (captopril 50 mg twice daily and valsartan 80 mg twice daily) in patients with a recent myocardial infarction (12 hours to 10 days) who exhibited clinical (70%) or radiologic (39%) evidence of heart failure or who had major LVSD (52%); 50% of patients fulfilled at least two sets of entry criteria. Patients with a systolic blood pressure <100 mmHg or serum creatinine >221 μmol/L were excluded. The focus in this section is on the outcome of combination therapy compared with either agent used alone.

Captopril was initiated at 6.25 mg twice daily and valsartan at 20 mg twice daily and rapid titration was encouraged prior to discharge. Measurement of serum potassium and creatinine was recommended during titration. Patients were monitored long term at 4-monthly intervals.

The primary end point was all-cause mortality and the principal secondary end point was a composite time-to-first event analysis of cardiovascular mortality, recurrent myocardial infarction, or hospitalization for heart failure.

A total of 14 703 patients were randomized and followed for a median of 24.7 months: 139 patients (<1%) were lost to follow-up; the mean age of the patients was 65 years old and 25% were aged ≥75 years old; most patients were men; 70% were taking a β-blocker at baseline but few were taking potassium sparing diuretics; 60% had an anterior myocardial infarction and 67% had a Q-wave infarction; 75% of patients were enrolled within 7 days of infarction. During this period, 46% underwent acute reperfusion therapy (thrombolysis or percutaneous intervention), 25% underwent late revascularization, and 17% had significant arrhythmias or conduction disturbances (mostly atrial fibrillation); 50% required treatment with diuretics. Of those randomized to valsartan alone, captopril, or the combination, 15.3%, 16.8%, and 19.0% had withdrawn from therapy by 12 months and the proportions taking target doses of therapy were 56%, 56%, and 47%, respectively. During the whole course of the study, 5.8%, 7.7%, and 9.0% of patients withdrew, respectively, from valsartan, captopril, or combination therapy for an adverse events and 20.5%, 21.6%, and 23.4% withdrew from therapy for any reason, most commonly patient choice for unspecified reasons. In each group, at 1 year, 7–8% were taking an open-label ACE inhibitor and 2–3% were taking an open-label ARB. Patients randomized to the combination were more likely to withdraw for hypotension (1.9% vs 0.8%) and renal dysfunction (1.3% vs 0.8%). Comparison of the adverse-effect profile of valsartan alone vs captopril is discussed below. Blood pressure rose during follow-up to a mean of 125/76 mmHg on captopril alone. Treatment with valsartan alone and in combination was associated with reductions in the rise of systolic blood pressures of 0.9 mmHg and 2.2 mmHg (both $p < 0.001$), respectively.

Mortality on combination therapy (19.3%) was similar to that on captopril alone (19.5%). The hazard ratio was 0.98, with 97.5% CIs of 0.89–1.09, which provided sufficient evidence to say that combination therapy was not inferior to captopril monotherapy. The proportions of patients reaching the principal secondary end point were also similar, at 31.1% on combination therapy and 31.9% on captopril alone. There was no interaction with β-blocker therapy. There was a trend for a reduction in the total number of investigator-defined hospital admissions for myocardial infarction or heart failure [estimated reduction of 15 (from 147 to 132) events per 1000 patients per year (NS)]. There was a trend to fewer recurrent hospitalizations on combination therapy.[94]

In summary, the reported data on this trial suggest that there is little advantage to using valsartan and captopril in combination compared with captopril alone. Combination therapy is associated with more adverse events and small health gains. However, data on symptoms have not yet been reported and could change the perceptions of the outcome of this study.

Overall, this group of trials suggests no effect of adding an ARB to an ACE inhibitor on mortality[81,82] (see Figure 9.6). The trials do suggest a symptomatic benefit, leading to a reduction in heart failure hospitalizations, which translates into an overall significant reduction in all-cause hospitalization.[81,82] These effects have generally been achieved despite the use of high background doses of ACE inhibitors. Although the benefits of adding an ARB to an ACE inhibitor might have been replicated by a substantial increase in the dose of the ACE inhibitor, there are few data to support this contention.[72] These results have been achieved with high doses of ARBs and it is not clear they can be replicated with lower doses.

Landmark trials principally designed to compare ARBs with ACE inhibitors (Tables 9.5–9.7; Figure 9.7)

This section includes the ELITE,[1] ELITE-II,[2,95] and OPTIMAAL studies.[25,26] The RESOLVD[3,82] and VALIANT[27,28,81] studies have complex designs, including a comparison of ARB against ACE inhibitor. Only a small amount of additional data can be gleaned from the meta-analyses of losartan and candesartan mentioned above and these are not dealt with further.

Table 9.5
Study design of and baseline characteristics of patients included in landmark trials of heart failure comparing ARB with ACE inhibitors.

	ELITE I[1]	ELITE II[2,95]
Comparison	Losartan vs captopril	Losartan vs captopril
n	722	3152
Mean follow-up (months)	11	18
Mean age (years)	74	71
≥70 years old (%) (entry criterion in brackets)	70 (≥65 years old)	– (≥60 years old)
Women (%)	33	30
NYHA (II/III/IV shown as %)	65/34/1	52/43/5
Mean LVEF (entry criterion in brackets)	31 (≤40%)	31 (≤40%)
Mean systolic blood pressure (mmHg) (entry criterion in brackets)	137 (>90 mmHg)	134 (>90 mmHg)
Cause of heart failure		
Ischemic heart disease	68	79
Other	32	21
Medical history		
Diabetes	25	24
Atrial fibrillation	23	30
Hypertension	57	49
Current angina	–	–
Pacemaker	–	–
Implantable defibrillator	–	–
CABG	–	–
Treatment		
Diuretic	74	78
ACE inhibitors	–	(prior to study 24%)
Beta-blockers	16	22
Potassium sparing diuretic	–	22
Calcium channel blocker	34	23
Digoxin	57	50
Anticoagulant	18	–
Aspirin	48	59
Statin	–	–

ELITE (Evaluation of Losartan In the Elderly Study)[1]

ELITE randomized 722 patients with heart failure and LVSD to captopril 50 mg three times a day or losartan 50 mg once daily in a double-blind study of 48 weeks' duration. The primary end point was an increase of serum creatinine of ≥26.5 μmol/L (0.3 mg/dl), which, as an index of an important adverse effect on renal function, appears arbitrary and unlikely to make most clinicians withdraw ACE inhibitor therapy or take any other action. The secondary end point,

Table 9.6
Summary of outcome of landmark trials of heart failure comparing ARB with an ACE inhibitor.

	Patients		Follow-up (months)	Mortality		Total no. of hospitalizations		Death or HF hospitalization: no. (%) of patients		Total HF hospitalizations	
	ACE inhibitor	ARB		ACE inhibitor	ARB	ACE inhibitor	ARB	ACE inhibitor	ARB	ACE inhibitor	ARB
ELITE I[1]	370	352	11	32	17	–	–	49 (13.2%)	33 (9.4%)	–	–
ELITE II[2]	1574	1578	18	250	280	–	–	–	–	–	–
Total for heart failure	**1944**	**1930**		**282 (14.5%)**	**297 (15.4%)**	–	–	–	–	–	–
OPTIMAAL[25,26]	2733	2744	32	447	499	Mean of 13.6 days	Mean of 13.1 days	–	–	–	–
VALIANT[4,27]	4909	4909	25	958	979	–	–	1335 (27.2%)	1326 (27.0%)	–	–
Total for myocardial infarction	**7642**	**7653**		**1405 (18.4%)**	**1478 (19.3%)**	–	–	–	–	–	–
Overall total	**9586**	**9583**		**1687 (17.6%)**	**1775 (18.5%)**	–	–	–	–	–	–

Table 9.7
Study design and baseline characteristics of patients included in landmark trials of ARBs in the setting of post-myocardial infarction, left ventricular systolic dysfunction, and/or heart failure.

	OPTIMAAL[25,26]	VALIANT[4,27,28]
Comparison	Losartan vs captopril	Valsartan vs captopril
n	5477	14 703
Mean follow-up (months)	32	25
Mean age (years)	67	65
>75 years old (%)	–	–
Women (%)	29	31
Killip class (I/II/III/IV shown as %)	32/57/9/2	29/48/17/6
Mean LVEF (entry criterion in brackets)	(<35% or new anterior Q-waves or heart failure)	35 (see text)
Mean systolic blood pressure (mmHg)	123 (>100 mmHg)	123 (>100 mmHg)
Time from infarction to randomization (median days)	3	5
Anterior site of infarction (%)	51	59
Medical history		
Prior myocardial infarction	18	28
Diabetes	17	23
Atrial fibrillation	10	
Hypertension	36	55
Any angioplasty/CABG*	14/3	35/7
Treatment		
Thrombolysis	54	35
Primary angioplasty	–	15
Diuretic	64	50
ACE inhibitors	Excluded	(40% prior to randomization)
Beta-blockers	79	70
Potassium sparing diuretic	–	9
Calcium channel blocker	22	–
Digoxin	11	–
Anticoagulant	–	–
Aspirin	96	91
Statin	31	34

*Includes acute revascularization prior to randomization.

death and/or admission for CHF, was formulated after patient recruitment was complete and after the results of other, smaller studies contained in the losartan meta-analysis had become known. Analyses of all-cause mortality and hospital admission for CHF were other pre-specified outcomes of interest and an analysis of all-cause hospital admission was conducted as a further exploratory analysis.

Patients had to be ≥65 years old and two-thirds were ≥70 years old. Patients were mostly in NYHA class II and only 74% of patients were receiving diuretics, a powerful stimulus to neuro-endocrine activation in heart failure, the substrate upon which ARBs and ACE inhibitors probably work. Over 80% of patients were in NYHA class I or II by the study end in both groups. The mean ejection fraction was 30%. Patients with renal dysfunction (serum creatinine ≥221 μmol/L (2.5 mg/dl) were excluded and thus a population at low risk of developing serious adverse renal events was identified. The mean baseline serum creatinine was 106 μmol/L (1.2 mg/dl). Compared to SOLVD treatment,[84] the ELITE population was about a decade older but appeared to have milder heart failure, as the ejection fraction was considerably higher and diuretic use was lower.

There was no difference in outcome with respect to changes in serum creatinine, with 10.5% of patients in each group having an increase ≥26.5 μmol/L. There was a trend to a greater increase in serum potassium with captopril, but it is not clear if this should be considered beneficial or not.

Losartan reduced overall mortality by 46% (RRR) ($p < 0.04$), largely due to a reduction in sudden deaths (RRR = 64%; $p < 0.05$) and death due to myocardial infarction (RRR = 76%; NS). Death due to progressive CHF occurred in only 1 patient in each group. Only 5.7% of patients in each group were hospitalized for CHF over 48 weeks, suggesting that the patients in ELITE had relatively mild CHF. Losartan and captopril exerted similar benefits on symptoms. Changes in plasma norepinephrine, a potential marker of progressive ventricular dysfunction, were not significantly different between groups.

Despite reducing mortality, which leaves more people at risk of hospitalization, losartan reduced all-cause hospitalization by 26% over and above any effect of captopril. This could have reflected the lower side-effect profile and better tolerability of losartan. Over 70% of patients were maintained on the target dose of both losartan and captopril, whereas 85% achieved the target dose at some time in the study. Overall, 20.8% of captopril-treated patients withdrew because of side effects vs 12.2% of losartan-treated patients ($p < 0.002$). This difference was largely due to a lower risk of cough, taste disturbance, angioedema, and worsening heart failure; 3.8% of patients discontinued captopril due to cough vs none on losartan ($p < 0.002$). There was no difference in the rate of hypotensive symptoms (24%).

Only when an effective drug is ingested can its benefits be realized. Thus, losartan could have proved superior to an ACE inhibitor not because it was more effective but because it was more likely to be taken. Excluding deaths, 18.2% of patients discontinued losartan for any reason vs 28.6% of those on captopril ($p < 0.001$), but this did not account for the difference in survival (3.7% vs 8.5% for those remaining on therapy with losartan or captopril, respectively; $p = 0.013$).

ELITE II[2,95]

ELITE II compared losartan (target dose 50 mg/day) with captopril (target dose 50 mg three times a day) in patients aged >60 years old with symptomatic heart failure and LVSD. By design, most patients had not previously received an ACE inhibitor or ARB. Patients with a systolic blood pressure <90 mmHg or serum creatinine >220 μmol/L were excluded. The primary end point was all-cause mortality. Losartan was initiated at 12.5 mg/day and captopril at 12.5 mg three times a day. Both were titrated at weekly intervals to target doses. Serum potassium and creatinine were measured regularly. Patients were monitored long term at 4-monthly intervals.

A total of 3152 patients were randomized and followed for a mean of 18 months. Only two patients were lost to follow-up. The mean age of the patients was 72 years old and 85% were aged ≥65 years old. Most patients were men and had coronary disease. Of those randomized to losartan, 23% were taking a β-blocker and 22% were taking a potassium-sparing diuretic. Adverse events led to withdrawal of study medication in about 10% and 15% of patients randomized to losartan and captopril, respectively. A large proportion of this difference was due to ACE inhibitor-induced cough. Losartan and captopril had similar effects on blood pressure.

There were slightly more deaths (absolute excess risk = 1.8%; relative excess risk = 13%; NS) on losartan compared with captopril. The confidence intervals (CIs) around this effect were sufficiently large that it is not safe to draw the conclusion that these drugs at these doses had equivalent effects. No significant differences were observed in rates of hospitalization for heart failure or other reasons. Patients taking β-blockers tended to fare better on captopril, although the statistical test for interaction (which is not a very powerful test) was not significant.

In summary, this trial does not support the substitution of an ACE inhibitor with losartan 50 mg/day in patients with heart failure. The previous ELITE study result appeared to have occurred by chance.

RESOLVD[3]

This study is reported in greater detail above. This section focuses on the comparison of ACE inhibitor and ARB; 327 patients were randomized to one of three doses of candesartan (4 mg, 8 mg, or 16 mg/day) or enalapril 20 mg/day. No differences in effect on symptoms, cardiac function, or neuroendocrine activation were observed. Patients on the two lower doses of candesartan tended to have higher mortality than patients on enalapril or the highest dose of candesartan. Differences in heart failure hospitalization favored enalapril. In summary, this trial is compatible with the ELITE II trial result but hints at the possibility that higher doses of ARBs may produce benefits similar to ACE inhibitors.

OPTIMAAL[25,26] *(see Tables 9.6 and 9.7)*

OPTIMAAL compared losartan (target dose 50 mg/day) with captopril (target dose 50 mg three times a day) in patients aged ≥50 years old with acute myocardial infarction and evidence of heart failure (81%) or major LVSD (LVEF <35% or end-diastolic dimension >65 mm (14%) or anterior Q-waves (51%)). Patients with a supine systolic blood pressure <100 mmHg or receiving an ACE inhibitor or ARB were excluded. The primary end point was all-cause mortality. Losartan was initiated at 12.5 mg/day and captopril at 6.25 mg (single dose), then 12.5 mg three times a day.

A total of 5477 patients were randomized and followed for a mean of 32 months. Only one patient was lost to follow-up. The mean age of the patients was 67 years old. Most patients were men and had coronary disease. Of those randomized to losartan, 79% were taking a β-blocker and 63% were taking a diuretic. Over 70% of patients had reached target doses of each drug at 1 month, rising to >80% by the end of the study. Adverse events led to withdrawal of study medication in 17% and 23% of patients randomized to losartan and captopril, respectively. A large proportion of this difference was due to ACE inhibitor-induced cough, but skin rashes, taste disturbances, and angioedema also made significant contributions. Losartan and captopril had similar effects on blood pressure in the long term, but captopril exerted a greater reduction after the first dose. Initiation of both agents was tolerated well.

There were slightly more deaths (absolute excess risk = 1.8%; relative excess risk = 13%; NS) on losartan compared with captopril. Despite the larger trial size and greater number of events, the CIs around this effect were still sufficiently large that a difference in mortality of up to 25% could not be excluded. No significant differences were observed in the risk of sudden death or resuscitated cardiac arrest or of myocardial infarction. There was no evidence of an interaction with β-blockers. Patients in both groups spent a similar number of days in hospital (about 13 days) and had similar severity of symptoms.

In summary, this trial does not support the substitution of an ACE inhibitor with losartan 50 mg/day in patients with post-infarction heart failure or ventricular dysfunction. These data are very similar to those observed in the ELITE II trial, except that they do not support a β-blocker interaction.

VALIANT[4,5,27,28,81] *(see Tables 9.6 and 9.7)*

This study is reported in greater detail above. This section focuses on the comparison of ACE inhibitor and ARB that included 4909 patients randomized to valsartan (160 mg twice daily) vs 4909 randomized to captopril (50 mg three times a day). Thus, the study had about twice as many patients in this head-to-head comparison compared with OPTIMAAL. Similar numbers of patients developed adverse events on captopril (28.4%) and valsartan (29.4%), although significantly fewer patients withdrew from valsartan because of side effects (7.7% vs 5.8%), although not for any reason (21.6% vs 20.5%). Hypotension (15.1% vs 11.9%), renal dysfunction (4.9% vs 3.0%) and withdrawal for hypotension (1.4% v 0.8%) were significantly more common with valsartan. Cough (5.0% vs 1.7%), rash (1.3% vs 0.7%), and taste disturbance (0.6% vs 0.3%) were all more common with captopril and more commonly led to withdrawal of therapy. Blood pressure rose during follow-up to a mean of 125/76 mmHg on captopril alone. Treatment with valsartan was associated with a reduction in this rise in systolic blood pressures of 0.9 mmHg ($p < 0.001$).

Mortality on valsartan (19.9%) was similar to that on captopril alone (19.5%). The hazard ratio was 1.00 with 97.5% CIs of 0.90–1.11, which provided sufficient evidence to say that valsartan was not inferior to captopril. The proportions of patients reaching the principal secondary end point were also similar, at 31.1% on valsartan and 31.9% on captopril. There was no interaction with β-blocker therapy. There was no difference in the total number of investigator-defined hospital admissions for myocardial infarction or heart failure.

In summary, the reported data on this trial suggest that valsartan and captopril provide similar benefits but that valsartan is associated with slightly fewer adverse events, although at increased cost.[94] This provides an argument for using an ARB in preference to an ACE inhibitor in this clinical setting, assuming that the cost of therapy, a very small fraction of overall health care, is not important.

In summary, these trials suggest that the benefits of treatment with an ACE inhibitor and an ARB, when prescribed in an adequate dose, are similar (see Table 9.6, Figure 9.7).[81,82] However, ARBs are associated with less adverse effects and therefore they could be considered the treatment of first choice. Although there are concerns that ARBs may exert less effect on reducing vascular events, this could reflect the use of inadequate doses. However, it is also possible that the full benefits of ACE inhibitors are not being observed due to the widespread use of aspirin, a treatment that has **not** been shown either to be effective in patients with heart failure or long term in patients who have had a myocardial infarction.[55,59] It is clear that aspirin reduces the benefits of ACE inhibitors[59,96] but may not reduce the benefits of ARBs.

Why use an ARB?

To improve symptoms of heart failure

There is good evidence that, compared with placebo, ARBs improve the symptoms of heart failure in patients with LVSD when used instead of ACE inhibitors.[13,14,78] There is good evidence that ARBs and ACE inhibitors improve symptoms to a similar extent.[97,98] ARBs also appear to improve symptoms compared with placebo when added to an ACE inhibitor,[4,13,14,20,78] although the latter effect appears modest, requiring treatment of 12–20 patients to improve 1 patient by 1 NYHA class compared with placebo. However, when the placebo effect is included, which corresponds better to the patient's experience, the effect may represent a substantial symptomatic benefit for 1 patient in 5.

The excess in adverse events should be set against the benefit on symptoms. Although the placebo-subtracted rate of withdrawal for adverse events is relatively low (2–5%), the absolute adverse event rate (more equivalent to the patient experience) may be 10–20%.

However, these assumptions do not account for the fact that patients were being closely monitored in a clinical trial and knew that the treatment might not work. Assuming that treatment is being recommended, the true benefits may be larger and adverse effects less than in the trial. Conversely, the inclusion of patients with more comorbidity may increase the adverse event rate.

There are insufficient data to evaluate the possible symptomatic benefits of ARBs in patients with heart failure and preserved left ventricular systolic function.

To reduce hospitalization

There is good evidence that, compared with placebo, ARBs reduce hospitalizations for worsening heart failure when used instead of ACE inhibitors and that this translates into a reduction in all-cause hospitalization.[6,75,81,82] There is fairly good evidence that ARBs and ACE inhibitors reduce hospitalizations to a similar extent.[2,25,95] There is also good evidence that ARBs reduce heart failure-related and all-cause hospitalization compared with placebo when added on top of an ACE inhibitor, and that the size of this effect is also similar to the effect observed in ACE inhibitor-naïve patients, suggesting that the benefits of treatment with this combination are additive.[8,81,82,90] In a recent meta-analysis, combination therapy reduced all-cause mortality or hospitalization for heart failure (odds ratio = 0.90; 0.82–0.99). Heart failure hospitalizations were reduced by about 20%, an effect that was large enough and robust enough to reduce all-cause hospitalization.[81,82]

The effects of ARBs on heart failure-related hospitalization in patients with preserved left ventricular systolic function were smaller and did not translate into a reduction in all-cause hospitalization, leaving some uncertainty about the true effect in this subset of patients.[10]

To reduce major vascular events

Unlike with ACE inhibitors,[39,85,86,99] there is little evidence that ARBs reduce the risk of myocardial infarction, although this must be viewed with caution in view of the ability of ARBs to reduce death in patients with heart failure, some of which are likely to have been vascular in origin. It is possible that ARBs and ACE inhibitors exert similar effects on vascular events, but that the effects are not additive. However, in CHARM-alternative there was no hint of a reduction in vascular events.[6] In studies of hypertension, ARBs appear effective in reducing stroke but also have not reduced the risk of myocardial infarction so far.[100] In studies of heart failure, ARBs have not reduced the risk of stroke. However, as in studies of hypertension, ARBs appear to retard or prevent the development of diabetes.[11]

To reduce mortality (Figures 9.3–9.5 and 9.7)

There is conclusive evidence that ARBs reduce mortality in patients with heart failure and LVSD in the absence of an ACE inhibitor.[6,75,81,82] In a recent meta-analysis of heart failure trials, ARBs reduced mortality by 20% compared with placebo (exact pooled odds ratio = 0.79, 95% CI = 0.66–0.94, without evidence of heterogeneity in outcome).[81,82] This is similar to the effect of ACE inhibitors compared with placebo in a recent meta-analysis (odds ratio = 0.83, 95% CI = 0.76–0.90).[101] Most but not all of these data are derived from studies of patients who have been intolerant of ACE inhibitors. However, although the data support, and it is rational to assume, that patients who can tolerate an ACE inhibitor would obtain similar benefits, due to the lack of evidence of an effect on vascular events in trials of heart failure or hypertension, some caution is still warranted. The magnitude of the effect is only similar to that observed with an ACE inhibitor when high doses of an ARB are used. When lower doses of ARB are used, there is evidence that they may be somewhat inferior to high-dose ACE inhibition, although dose-ranging studies of ACE inhibitors themselves have not shown a clear dose–response against mortality. Also, ACE inhibitors appear to be disadvantaged by non-evidenced-based therapy with aspirin and their benefits may be greater if such treatment is eliminated.[55,59,96]

In the presence of an ACE inhibitor, the overall data suggest no mortality benefit from combination therapy compared with an ACE inhibitor only (odds ratio = 1.08, 0.62–2.60) in trials of heart failure and left ventricular systolic dysfunction.[4,8,81,82] There is no evidence of a mortality benefit in patients with heart failure and preserved LV systolic function.

Adverse effects

A persistent dry cough is undoubtedly a side effect of ACE inhibitors, especially among women.[6,7,102] However, the amount of disability it causes is unclear. Cough is reported spontaneously as an adverse effect in studies of ACE inhibitors in about 3–5% of cases, little higher than with placebo.[99,103] Some patients have a severe cough due to ACE inhibitors, but, surprisingly, even if severe, do not report it spontaneously, believing the side effect to be part of their illness. Cough can be disabling, physically tiring the patient and disrupting sleep; undoubtedly, some patients 'cough themselves to death'. Cough does not appear to be a side effect of ARBs. Recurrence of cough when patients are switched from an ACE inhibitor to an ARB is unlikely and should provoke investigation to exclude lung pathology or gastro-oesophageal reflux. Cough was reported as a side effect of ACE inhibitors in 5% of patients in

VALIANT and 18.7% in OPTIMAAL; respective data for ARBs were 1.7% and 9.3%. Patients were rarely withdrawn for cough on an ARB compared with an ACE inhibitor (2.5% vs 0.6% in VALIANT and 4.1% vs 1.0% in OPTIMAAL).

The mechanism underlying ACE inhibitor-induced cough is unclear but may include effects on pulmonary bradykinin or on mast cells.[104–107] Switching ACE inhibitors occasionally helps, but this may have more to do with the interruption of therapy than real differences between ACE inhibitors. Anecdotally, ACE inhibitors may perpetuate cough due to a respiratory tract infection; a drug-free interval may be all that is necessary to stop the cough, the patient then being able to resume the same treatment. Switching patients who cough from ACE inhibitors to ARBs seems a safe and reliable way to avoid cough.

Angioneurotic edema

Clinical trials of CHF have suggested that this side effect of ACE inhibitors is rare and certainly <1%.[6,7,99,103] The mechanism underlying this reaction is also unclear but may be mediated by bradykinin and mast cells. Patients on renal dialysis are at greater risk of angioneurotic reactions.[108] ARBs have not been shown to precipitate more angioneurotic reactions than a placebo.

Hypotension

Serious hypotension was generally no more common with ARB than with ACE inhibitor mono-therapy in the above trials. There is a slight increase in hypotensive problems when ACE inhibitors and ARBs are used in combination, one indication that the ARB is having an additive effect.[8] Patients who do not tolerate an ACE inhibitor because of hypotension will commonly not tolerate an ARB.[7,109] Initial doses of either may precipitate acute hypotension, indicating that patients should be started on small doses and that patients on large doses of diuretic or with a low arterial pressure should be observed for a few hours after the initial dose.[34,70,110–112] The existing data provided in the studies need to be interpreted with caution because they generally fail to distinguish clearly between syncope, a hemodynamic crisis, and symptomless hypotension.

Renal dysfunction

Renal dysfunction is most likely to occur when ACE inhibitors are given to very elderly patients (age >75 years old), patients with severe CHF, and those with pre-existing renal disease. No differences in the effects of ACE inhibitors and ARBs on renal function in heart failure have been noted so far.[1] However, it is likely that patient selection excluded many patients at increased risk for renal dysfunction. Addition of an ARB to an ACE inhibitor may double the risk of the need to withdraw therapy due to worsening renal function (from 4.1% to 7.8% in

CHARM-added; 0.2% to 1.1% in Val-HeFT).[4,8] ARBs, like ACE inhibitors, appear to reduce proteinuria and retard the long-term decline in renal function in non-heart failure patients.[113–115] The significance of the uricosuric effect of losartan, an effect that may not be shared with other ARBs, is uncertain.[66]

Are the benefits and side effects of ARBs dose-related? (Table 9.8)

Studies investigating a dose–response in hemodynamics, neuroendocrine effects, and effects on ventricular function and remodeling and on symptoms and exercise capacity, all suggest a dose–response but have not convincingly shown where the top of the dose–response lies.[3,70,116] It is notable that in CHARM, the most successful ARB study so far, the target dose was double the highest dose used in any published dose–response study with this agent. In contrast, there is limited evidence of a dose–response in terms of death or hospitalization in dose–response studies. However, the failure of lower doses of losartan to have equivalent effects to high-dose captopril,[2,25,115] and the magnitude of the effect of high-dose candesartan in CHARM implies that larger doses may be more effective. The HEAL study, comparing losartan 50 mg/day with 150 mg/day in patients with heart failure who are ACE intolerant, may provide some insights.

Are there clinically relevant differences between ARBs?

The evidence is consistent with a class effect so far. Possible differences in outcome appear to owe more to differences in dose. Pharmacokinetic differences may dictate how often the treatment should be given. The possible different effect of losartan on uricosuria is of uncertain significance. Studies of hypertension suggest that there may be differences in potency between ARBs,[117] with the maximum blood pressure reduction that can be achieved with losartan being about 3 mmHg less than that achieved with candesartan.

Are there important interactions between ARBs and other classes of drug used in heart failure?

The CHARM program suggested no interaction with background therapy.[9] Of note, earlier concerns about a potential interaction with β-blockers were laid to rest.[8,9] However, a potential synergistic interaction between β-blockers and ACE inhibitors that is absent with ARBs cannot be discounted.

ARBs increase the risk of hyperkalemia and therefore there is a potential for an adverse interaction with aldosterone antagonists. Relatively few patients ($n = 1272$) were taking spironolactone in CHARM and only 437 patients were in the CHARM-added trial.[9] Trends to less effect in this subgroup of patients were not significant in the overall analysis, but more data

Table 9.8
Dose–response studies with ARBs in CHF and clinical outcome.*

Drugs and references					
Losartan[70] (n = 134)	Dose (mg)	Placebo	2.5	10	25	50
	Worsening (%)	26	NR†	20	10	9
	Improvement (%)	NR	NR	NR	48	52
Irbesartan[116] (n = 218)	Dose (mg)	Not studied	12.5	37.5	75	150
	Discontinuation for worsening (%)	Not studied	9.3	11.1	3.6	1.8
Candesartan (RESOLVD)[3] (n = 768)	Dose (mg)	Enalapril	4	8	16	Combination
	Death (%)	3.7	6.3	7.4	4.6	8.7
	Death or CHF hospitalization (%)	9.2	15.3	20.4	14.8	17.5
Candesartan (STRETCH)[78] (n = 926)	Dose (mg)	Placebo	—	4	8	16
	Symptoms and exercise capacity	—	—	Improvement in symptoms with all doses of candesartan compared with placebo. Dose-related improvement in exercise capacity		

*Trends to prevention of worsening with higher doses were not statistically significant in the studies with losartan and irbesartan.
†NR, not reported.

on the safety and utility of quadruple therapy with ACE inhibitors, β-blockers, aldosterone antagonists, and ARBs are required.

There is strong evidence for an adverse interaction on mortality between ACE inhibitors, but not ARBs, and aspirin.[55–60,99] In addition, one small ($n = 16$) cross-over study with 3-week treatment periods suggested that the improvement in exercise capacity with losartan but not enalapril could be inhibited by aspirin.[118]

Heart failure in the absence of left ventricular systolic dysfunction

The CHARM-preserved study provides weak support for the use of an ARB in patients with heart failure and preserved LVSD. The small observed benefit may be due to improved control of blood pressure. There are few supportive data. Warner et al[119] performed a randomized, double-blind, placebo-controlled, cross-over study of 2 weeks of losartan (50 mg/day) with a 2-week washout period on 20 patients with normal LV systolic function (EF >55%), no evidence of ischemia, a mitral flow velocity E/A < 1, normal resting SBP (<150 mmHg), but a hypertensive response to exercise (SBP >200 mmHg). The primary outcome measures were exercise tolerance and quality of life. After 2 weeks of losartan, peak SBP during exercise decreased by 30 mmHg ($p < 0.01$), and exercise time increased by about 60 seconds compared with placebo. Quality of life improved with losartan compared with baseline and placebo.

Conclusions

ARBs are a substantial step forward in the treatment of heart failure; they are superior to placebo in improving symptoms, morbidity, and mortality in patients with CHF who are intolerant of ACE inhibitors or who have contraindications to them. It seems likely that adequate doses of ARBs are as effective as ACE inhibitors and their tolerability profile is impressive. In women, in whom the incidence of ACE inhibitor cough is high, and in patients with a history of multiple allergies or on renal dialysis that could predispose to angioedema, some might consider ARBs as the initial treatment of choice. However, the lack of evidence for an effect on coronary vascular events raises the possibility that all the benefits of ACE inhibitors are not replicated by ARBs and that activation of the bradykinin–prostaglandin pathway is an important mechanism of ACE inhibitor benefit, although potentially attenuated by the use of aspirin.

ARBs do not reduce mortality when added to an ACE inhibitor but do improve symptoms and reduce hospitalization. The benefits appear sufficiently large that such treatment can be advised in many patients, especially those at highest risk of such events. Health economic analyses of cost-effectiveness are awaited.

The data on heart failure with preserved LV systolic function are insufficient to make any strong recommendation. Greater understanding of this population and focus on subgroups with increased risk (for instance those with increased brain natriuretic peptide) or that have a substrate upon which ARBs are likely to work (hypertension) may increase the benefits obtained.

References

1. Pitt B, Segal R, Martinez FA et al, on behalf of the ELITE study group. Randomised trial of losartan versus captopril in patients over 65 with heart failure (Evaluation of losartan in the elderly study, ELITE). Lancet 1997; 349:747–52.
2. Pitt B, Poole Wilson PA, Segal R et al, on behalf of the ELITE II investigators. Effect of losartan compared with captopril on mortality in patients with symptomatic heart failure: randomised trial – the Losartan Heart Failure Survival Study ELITE II. Lancet 2000; 355:1582–7.
3. McKelvie RS, Yusuf S, Pericak D et al. Comparison of candesartan, enalapril and their combination in congestive heart failure. Randomized evaluation of strategies for left ventricular dysfunction (RESOLVD) Pilot Study. Circulation 1999; 100(10):1056–64.
4. Cohn JN, Tognoni G, for the Valsartan Heart Failure Trial Investigators. A randomized trial of the angiotensin-receptor blocker valsartan in chronic heart failure. N Engl J Med 2001; 345(23):1667–75.
5. Cohn JN, Tognoni G, Glazer RD, Spormann D. Baseline demographics of the valsartan heart failure trial. Eur J Heart Failure 2000; 2:439–46.
6. Granger CB, McMurray JJV, Yusuf S et al, for the CHARM Investigators and Committees. Effects of candesartan in patients with chronic heart failure and reduced left-ventricular systolic function intolerant to angiotensin-converting-enzyme inhibitors: the CHARM-Alternative trial. Lancet 2003; 362:772–6.
7. McMurray J, Ostergren J, Pfeffer M et al, on behalf of the CHARM Committees and Investigators. Clinical features and contemporary management of patients with low and preserved ejection fraction heart failure: baseline characteristics of patients in the Candesartan in Heart failure – Assessment of Reduction in Mortality and morbidity (CHARM) programme. Eur J Heart Failure 2003; 5:261–70.
8. McMurray JJV, Ostergren J, Swedberg K et al, for the CHARM Investigators and Committees. Effects of candesartan in patients with chronic heart failure and reduced left-ventricular systolic function taking angiotensin-converting-enzyme inhibitors: the CHARM-Added trial. Lancet 2003; 362:767–71.
9. Pfeffer MA, Swedberg K, Granger CB et al, for the CHARM Investigators and Committees. Effects of candesartan on mortality and morbidity in patients with chronic heart failure; the CHARM-Overall programme. Lancet 2003; 362:759–66.
10. Yusuf S, Pfeffer MA, Swedberg K et al, for the CHARM Investigators and Committees. Effects of candesartan in patients with chronic heart failure and preserved left-ventricular ejection fraction: the CHARM-Preserved Trial. Lancet 2003; 362:771–81.
11. Yusuf S, Ostergren J, Gerstein HC et al, on behalf of the Candesartan in Heart Failure – Assessment of Reduction in Mortality and Morbidity Program (CHARM) Investigators. Effects of candesartan on the development of a new diagnosis of diabetes mellitus in patients with heart failure. Circulation 2005; 112(48):53.
12. Solomon SD, Wang D, Finn P et al. Effect of candesartan on cause-specific mortality in heart failure patients. The Candesartan in Heart failure Assessment of Reduction in Mortality and morbidity (CHARM) program. Circulation 2004; 110:2180–3.
13. O'Meara E, Solomon S, McMurray J et al. Effect of candesartan on New York Heart Association functional class. Eur Heart J 2004; 25:1920–6.
14. O'Meara E, Lewis E, Granger C et al. Patient perception of the effect of treatment with candesartan in heart failure. Results of the Candesartan in Heart failure: Assessment of Reduction in Mortality and morbidity (CHARM) programme. Eur J Heart Fail 2005; 7:650–6.
15. Maggioni AP, Opasich C, Anand I et al. Anemia in patients with heart failure: prevalence and prognostic role in a controlled trial and in clinical practice. J Card Fail 2005; 11(2):91–8.

16. Anand I, Kuskowski MA, Rector TS et al, for the Val-HeFT Investigators. Anemia and change in hemoglobin over time related to mortality and morbidity in patients with chronic heart failure: results from Val-HeFT. Circulation 2005; 112:1121–7.

17. Anand IS, Latini R, Florea VG et al, for the Val-HeFT Investigators. C-reactive protein in heart failure: prognostic value and the effect of valsartan. Circulation 2005; 112:1428–34.

18. Baruch L, Glazer RD, Aknay N et al. Morbidity, mortality, physiologic and functional parameters in elderly and non-elderly patients in the Valsartan Heart Failure Trial (Val-HeFT). Am Heart J 2004; 148:951–7.

19. Krum H, Carson P, Farsang C et al. Effect of valsartan added to background ACE inhibitor therapy in patients with heart failure: results from Val-HeFT. Eur J Heart Fail 2004; 6:937–45.

20. Majani G, Giardini A, Opasich C et al. Effect of valsartan on quality of life when added to usual therapy for heart failure: results from the Valsartan Heart Failure Trial. J Card Fail 2005; 11(4):253–9.

21. Maggioni AP, Latini R, Carson PE et al. Valsartan reduces the incidence of atrial fibrillation in patients with heart failure: results from the Valsartan Heart Failure Trial (Val-HeFT). Am Heart J 2005; 149:548–57.

22. Demers C, McMurray JJ, Swedberg K et al, CHARM Investigators. Impact of candesartan on nonfatal myocardial infarction and cardiovascular death in patients with heart failure. JAMA 2005; 294:1794–8.

23. Sharma D, Buyse M, Pitt B, Rucinska EJ, and the Losartan Heart Failure Morbidity Meta-analysis Study Group. Meta-analysis of observed mortality data from all controlled, double-blind multiple-dose studies of losartan in heart failure. Am J Cardiol 2000; 85:187–92.

24. Erdmann E, George M, Voet B et al. The safety and tolerability of candesartan cilexetil in CHF. J Renin Angiotensin Aldosterone Syst 2000; 1(Suppl 1):31–6.

25. Dickstein K, Kjekshus J, and the OPTIMAAL Steering Committee for the OPTIMAAL Study Group. Effects of losartan and captopril on mortality and morbidity in high-risk patients after acute myocardial infarction: the OPTIMAAL randomised trial. Lancet 2002; 360:752–60.

26. Dickstein K, Kjekshus J, for the OPTIMAAL Trial Steering Committee and Investigators. Comparison of baseline data, initial course and management: losartan versus captopril following acute myocardial infarction (The OPTIMAAL Trial). Am J Cardiol 2001; 87:766–71.

27. Pfeffer MA, McMurray JJ, Velazquez EJ et al, for the Valsartan in Acute Myocardial Infarction Trial Investigators. Valsartan, captopril, or both in myocardial infarction complicated by heart failure, left ventricular dysfunction, or both. N Engl J Med 2003; 349:1893–906.

28. Velazquez EJ, Pfeffer MA, McMurray JJV et al. VALsartan In Acute myocardial iNfarcTion (VALIANT) trial: baseline characteristics in context. Eur J Heart Fail 2003; 5:537–44.

29. Cleland JGF, Witte K, Thackray S. Bradykinin and ventricular function. Eur Heart J 2000; Suppl H(2):H20–9.

30. Zusman RM. Effects of converting-enzyme inhibitors on the renin–angiotensin–aldosterone, bradykinin, and arachidonic acid–prostaglandin systems: correlation of chemical structure and biological activity. Am J Kidney Dis 1987; 10:13–23.

31. Cleland JGF, Dargie HJ, Hodsman GP et al. Captopril in heart failure. A double blind controlled trial. Br Heart J 1984; 52(530):535.

32. Cleland JGF, Semple P, Hodsman GP et al. Angiotensin II levels, haemodynamics and sympathoadrenal function after low-dose captopril in heart failure. Am J Med 1984; 77:880–6.

33. Cleland JGF, Dargie HJ, Ball SG et al. Effects of enalapril in heart failure: a double blind study of effects on exercise performance, renal function, hormones and metabolic state. Br Heart J 1985; 54:305–12.

34. Cleland JGF, Dargie HJ, McAlpine H et al. Severe hypotension after first dose of enalapril in heart failure. BMJ 1985; 291:1309–12.

35. Cleland JGF, Dargie HJ, East BW et al. Total body and serum electrolyte composition in heart failure: The effects of captopril. Eur Heart J 1985; 6:681–8.

36. Cleland JGF, Dargie HJ. Heart failure, renal function, and angiotensin converting enzyme inhibitors. Kidney Int 1987; 31:S220–8.

37. Cleland JGF, Gillen G, Dargie HJ. The effects of frusemide and angiotensin-converting enzyme inhibitors and their combination on cardiac and renal haemodynamics in heart failure. Eur Heart J 1988; 9(2):132–41.

38. Cleland JGF, Krikler D. Modification of atherosclerosis by agents that do not lower cholesterol. Br Heart J 1993; 69:54–62.

39. Lonn EM, Yusuf S, Jha P et al. Emerging role of angiotensin converting enzyme inhibitors in cardiac and vascular protection. Circulation 1994; 90:2056–69.

40. Minisi AJ, Thames MD. Distribution of left ventricular sympathetic afferents demonstrated by reflex responses to transmural myocardial ischaemia and to intracoronary and epicardial bradykinin. Circulation 1993; 87:240–6.

41. Morgan K, Wharton J, Webb JC et al. Co-expression of renin–angiotensin system component genes in human atrial tissue. J Hypertens 1994; 12(Suppl 4):S11–19.

42. Cleland JGF, Cowburn PJ, Morgan K. Neuroendocrine activation after myocardial infarction: causes and consequences. Heart 1996; 76(Suppl 3):53–9.

43. Johnston CI, Risvanis J. Preclinical pharmacology of angiotensin II receptor antagonists. Am J Hypertens 1997; 10:306–10S.

44. Smith RD, Timmermans C. Human angiotensin receptor subtypes. Curr Opinion Nephrol Hypertens 1994; 3:112–22.

45. Timmermans PB, Benfield P, Chiu AT et al. Angiotensin II receptors and functional correlates. Am J Hypertens 1992; 5:221–35S.

46. Asano K, Dutcher DL, Port JD et al. Selective downregulation of the angiotensin II AT-1-receptor subtype in failing human ventricular myocardium. Circulation 1997; 95:1193–200.

47. Haywood GA, Gullestad L, Katsuya T et al. AT-1 and AT-2 angiotensin receptor gene expression in human heart failure. Circulation 1997; 95:1201–6.

48. Regitz-Zagrosek V, Friedel N, Heymann A et al. Regulation of the angiotensin receptor subtypes in cell cultures, animal models and human diseases. Circulation 1995; 91:1461–71.

49. Stoll M, Stecklings UM, Paul M et al. The angiotensin AT2-receptor mediates inhibition of cell proliferation in coronary endothelial cells. J Clin Invest 1995; 95:651–7.

50. Yamada T, Akishita M, Pollman MJ et al. Angiotensin II type 2 receptor mediates vascular smooth muscle cell apoptosis and antagonizes angiotensin II type I receptor action: an in vitro gene transfer study. Life Sci 1998; 63:PL289–95.

51. Pitt B. 'Escape' of aldosterone production in patients with left ventricular dysfunction treated with an angiotensin converting enzyme inhibitor: implications for therapy. Cardiovasc Drugs Ther 1995; 9(1):145–9.

52. MacFadyen RJ, Lee AFC, Morton JJ, Pringle SD, Struthers AD. How often are angiotensin II and aldosterone concentrations raised during chronic ACE inhibitor treatment in cardiac failure? Heart 1999; 82(1):57–61.

53. Struthers AD, Anderson G, MacFadyen RJ, Fraser C, MacDonald TM. Non-adherence with ACE inhibitor treatment is common in heart failure and can be detected by routine serum ACE activity assays. Heart 1999; 82:584–8.

54. Teo K, Yusuf S, Pfeffer M, Kober L et al, for the ACE Inhibitors Collaborative Group. Effects of long-term treatment with angiotensin-converting-enzyme inhibitors in the presence or absence of aspirin: a systematic review. Lancet 2002; 360:1037–43.

55. Cleland JGF, Bulpitt CJ, Falk RH et al. Is aspirin safe for patients with heart failure? Br Heart J 1995; 74(3):215–19.

56. Cleland JGF, John J, Houghton T. Does aspirin attenuate the effect of angiotensin-converting enzyme inhibitors in hypertension or heart failure? Curr Opin Nephrol Hypertens 2001; 10:625–31.

57. Cleland JGF. No reduction in cardiovascular risk with NSAIDs – including aspirin? Lancet 2002; 359(9301):92–3.

58. Cleland JGF. For debate: preventing atherosclerotic events with aspirin. BMJ 2002; 324(7329):103–5.

59. Cleland JGF. Is aspirin 'the weakest link' in cardiovascular prophylaxis. The surprising lack of evidence supporting the use of aspirin for cardiovascular disease. Prog Cardiovasc Dis 2002; 44:275–92.

60. Cleland JGF. Anticoagulant and antiplatelet therapy in heart failure. Curr Opin Cardiol 1997; 12:276–87.

61. Herrlin B, Nyquist O, Sylven C. Induction of a reduction in haemoglobin concentration by enalapril in stable, moderate heart failure: a double blind study. Br Heart J 1991; 66(3):199–205.

62. Belcher G, Hubner R, George M, Elmfeldt D, Lunde H. Candesartan cilexetil: safety and tolerability in healthy volunteers and patients with hypertension. J Hum Hypertens 1997; 11(Suppl 2):S85–9.

63. Brooksby P, Robinson PJ, Segal R et al. Effects of losartan and captopril on QT-dispersion in elderly patients with heart failure. ELITE study group. Lancet 1999; 354:395–6.

64. Binkley PF, Haas GJ, Starling RC et al. Sustained augmentation of parasympathetic tone with angiotensin-converting enzyme inhibition in patients with congestive heart failure. J Am Coll Cardiol 1993; 21:655–61.

65. Binkley PF, Nunziata E, Leier CV. Selective AT-1 blockade with losartan does not restore autonomic balance in patients with heart failure. J Am Coll Cardiol 1998; 31(Suppl A): 250A.

66. Wurzner G, Gerster JC, Chiolero A et al. Comparative effects of losartan and irbesartan on serum uric acid in hypertensive patients with hyperuricaemia and gout. J Hypertens 2001; 19:1855–60.

67. Puig JG, Torres R, Ruilope LM. AT1 blockers and uric acid metabolism: are there relevant differences? J Hypertens 2002; 20(Suppl 5):S29–31.

68. Leyva F, Anker S, Swan JW. Serum uric acid as an index of impaired oxidative metabolism in chronic heart failure. Eur Heart J 1997; 18:858–65.

69. Bloom BS. Continuation of antihypertensive medication after 1 year of therapy. Clin Ther 1998; 20:671–81.

70. Crozier I, Ikram H, Awan N et al. Losartan in heart failure: hemodynamic effects and tolerability. Circulation 1995; 91:691–7.

71. Pitt B, Dickstein K, Benedict C et al. The randomized angiotensin receptor antagonist – ACE inhibitor study (RAAS) – pilot study. Circulation 1996; 94(Suppl):I-428.

72. Packer M, Poole Wilson PA, Armstrong PW et al, on behalf of the ATLAS investigators. Comparative effects of low and high doses of the angiotensin-converting enzyme inhibitor, lisinopril, on morbidity and mortality in chronic heart failure. Circulation 1999; 100:2312–18.

73. The NETWORK Investigators. Clinical outcome with enalapril in symptomatic chronic heart failure; a dose comparison. Eur Heart J 1998; 19:481–9.

74. Cleland JGF, Poole-Wilson PA. ACE inhibitors for heart failure: a question of dose. Br Heart J 1994; 72:106–10.

75. Maggioni A, Anand I, Gottlieb SO et al, for the Valsartan Heart Failure Trial Investigators. Effects of valsartan on morbidity and mortality in patients with heart failure not receiving angiotensin converting enzyme inhibitors. J Am Coll Cardiol 2002; 40:1414–21.

76. Banerjee P, Banerjee T, Khand A, Clark AL, Cleland JGF. Diastolic heart failure – neglected or misdiagnosed? J Am Coll Cardiol 2002; 39(1):138–41.

77. Klinge R, Polis A, Dickstein K, Hall C. Effects of angiotensin II receptor blockade on N-terminal proatrial natriuretic factor plasma levels in chronic heart failure. J Card Fail 1997; 3:75–81.

78. Riegger GAJ, Bouzo H, Petr P et al, for the STRETCH Investigators. Improvement in exercise tolerance and symptoms of congestive heart failure during treatment with candesartan cilexetil. Circulation 1999; 100:2224–30.

79. Bart BA, Ertl G, Held P et al. Contemporary management of patients with left ventricular systolic dysfunction. Results from the Study of Patients Intolerant of Converting Enzyme Inhibitors (SPICE) Registry. Eur Heart J 1999; 20(16):1182–90.

80. Matsumori A. Efficacy and safety of oral candesartan cilexetil in patients with congestive heart failure. Eur J Heart Fail 2003; 5(5):669–77.

81. Cleland JGF, Freemantle N, Kaye GC et al. Clinical trials update from the American Heart Association: omega-3 fatty acids and arrhythmia risk in patients with implantable defibrillators, ACTIV in CHF, VALIANT, the Hanover autologous bone marrow transplantation study, SPORTIF V, ORBIT and PAD and DEFINITE. Eur J Heart Fail 2004; 6:109–15.

82. Coletta AP, Cleland JGF, Freemantle N et al. Clinical trials update from the European Society of Cardiology: CHARM, BASEL, EUROPA and ESTEEM. Eur J Heart Fail 2003; 5(5):697–704.

83. Swedberg K, Pfeffer M, Granger C et al, for the CHARM-Programme Investigators. Candesartan in heart failure – assessment of reduction in mortality and morbidity (CHARM): rationale and design. J Card Fail 1999; 5(3):276–82.

84. Yusuf S. Effect of enalapril on survival in patients with reduced left ventricular ejection fractions and congestive heart failure. N Engl J Med 1991; 325:293–302.

85. The Heart Outcomes Prevention Evaluation Study Investigators. Effects of angiotensin-converting-enzyme inhibitor, ramipril, on cardiovascular events in high risk patients. N Engl J Med 2000; 342:145–53.

86. The EURopean trial On reduction of cardiac events with Perindopril in stable coronary Artery disease Investigators. Efficacy of perindopril in reduction of cardiovascular events among patients with stable coronary artery disease: randomised, double-blind, placebo-controlled, multicentre trial (the EUROPA study). Lancet 2003; 362:782–8.

87. Cleland JGF, Swedberg K, Follath F et al, for the Study Group on Diagnosis of the Working Group on Heart Failure of the European Society of Cardiology. The EuroHeart Failure survey programme – a survey on the quality of care among patients with heart failure in Europe. Part 1: patient characteristics and diagnosis. Eur Heart J 2003; 24:422–63.

88. Cleland JGF, Tendera M, Adamus J et al, on behalf of the PEP-CHF Investigators. Perindopril for elderly people with chronic heart failure: the PEP-CHF study. Eur J Heart Fail 1999; 1:211–17.

89. Anand IS, Fisher LD, Chiang Y-T et al, for the Val-HeFT Investigators. Changes in brain natriuretic peptide and norepinephrine over time and mortality and morbidity in the Valsartan Heart Failure Trial (Val-HeFT). Circulation 2003; 107:1278–83.

90. Carson P, Tognoni G, Cohn JN. Effect of valsartan on hospitalization: results from Val-HeFT. J Card Fail 2003; 9:164–71.

91. Latini R, Masson S, Anand I et al, for the Val-HeFT Investigators. Effects of valsartan on circulating brain natriuretic peptide and norepinephrine in symptomatic chronic heart failure: the Valsartan Heart Failure Trial (Val-HeFT). Circulation 2002; 106:2454–8.

92. Wong M, Staszewsky L, Latini R et al. Valsartan benefits left ventricular structure and function in heart failure: Val-HeFT echocardiographic study. J Am Coll Cardiol 2002; 40(5):970–5.

93. Cohn JN, Tognoni G, Glazer RD, Spormann D, Hester A. Rationale and design of the valsartan heart failure trial: a large multinational trial to assess the effects of valsartan, an angiotensin-receptor blocker, on morbidity and mortality in chronic congestive heart failure. J Card Fail 1999; 5:155–60.

94. Reed SD, Radeva JI, Weinfurt KP et al, VALIANT Investigators. Resource use, costs, and quality of life among patients in the multinational Valsartan in Acute Myocardial Infarction Trial (VALIANT). Am Heart J 2005; 150:323–9.

95. Pitt B, Poole-Wilson PA, Segal R et al. Effects of losartan versus captopril on mortality in patients with symptomatic heart failure: rationale, design and baseline characteristics of patients in the Losartan Heart Failure Survival Study – ELITE II. J Card Fail 1999; 5:146–54.

96. Teo KK, Yusuf S, Pfeffer M, ACE Inhibitors Collaborative Group. Effects of long-term treatment with ACE inhibitors in the presence or absence of aspirin: a systematic review. Lancet 2002; 360:1037–43.

97. Dickstein K, Chang P, Willenheimer R et al. Comparison of the effects of losartan and enalapril on clinical status and exercise performance in patients with moderate or severe chronic heart failure. J Am Coll Cardiol 1995; 26(2):438–45.

98. Lang RM, Elkayam U, Yellen LG et al, on behalf of the Losartan Pilot Exercise Study Investigators. Comparative effects of losartan and enalapril on exercise capacity and clinical status in patients with heart failure. J Am Coll Cardiol 1997; 30:983–91.

99. Yusuf S. Effect of enalapril on survival in patients with reduced left ventricular ejection fractions and congestive heart failure. N Engl J Med 1991; 325:293–302.

100. Dahlof B, Devereux RB, Kjeldsen SE et al. Cardiovascular morbidity and mortality in the losartan intervention for endpoint reduction in hypertension study (LIFE): a randomised trial against atenolol. Lancet 2002; 359:995–1003.

101. Eccles M, Freemantle N, Mason JM, for the North of England Evidence Based Guideline Development Project. Evidence based clinical practice guideline: ACE inhibitors in the primary care management of adults with symptomatic heart failure. BMJ 1998; 316:1369–75.

102. Os I, Bratland B, Dahlof B et al. Female sex as an important determinant of lisinopril-induced cough. Lancet 1992; 339:303–10.

103. Kostis JB, Shelton B, Gosselin G et al. Adverse effects of enalapril in the Studies of Left Ventricular Dysfunction (SOLVD). Am Heart J 1996; 131:350–5.

104. Israili ZH, Hall WD. Cough and angioneurotic edema associated with angiotensin-converting enzyme inhibitor therapy. A review of the literature and pathophysiology. Ann Intern Med 1992; 117:234–42.

105. Malini PL, Strocchi E, Zanardi M, Milani M, Ambrosioni E. Thromboxane antagonism and cough induced by angiotensin-converting enzyme inhibitor. Lancet 1997; 350:15–18.

106. Cleland JGF. Lack of effect of nedocromil sodium in ACE inhibitor-induced cough. Lancet 1995; 345:394.

107. Hargreaves MR, Benson MK. Inhaled sodium cromoglycate in angiotensin converting enzyme inhibitor induced cough. Lancet 1995; 345:13–16.

108. Schulman G, Hakim R, Arias R et al. Bradykinin generation by dialysis membranes: possible role in anaphylactic reaction. J Am Soc Nephrol 1993; 3:1563–9.

109. Granger CB, Ertl G, Kuch J et al. Randomized trial of candesartan cilexetil in the treatment of patients with congestive heart failure and a history of intolerance to angiotensin-converting enzyme inhibitors. Am Heart J 2000; 139(4):609–17.

110. Gottlieb SS, Dickstein K, Fleck E et al. Hemodynamic and neurohormonal effects of the angiotensin II antagonist losartan in patients with congestive heart failure. Circulation 1993; 88:1602–9.

111. Cleland J, Semple P, Hodsman P et al. Angiotensin II levels, hemodynamics, and sympathoadrenal function after low dose captopril in heart failure. Am J Med 1984; 77:880–6.

112. Kostis J, Shelton BJ, Yusuf S et al. Tolerability of enalapril by patients with left ventricular dysfunction: results of the medication challenge phase of the studies of left ventricular dysfunction. Am Heart J 1994; 128:358–64.

113. Mogensen CE, Neldam S, Tikkanen I et al, for the CALM Study Group. Randomised controlled trial of dual blockade of renin–angiotensin system in patients with hypertension, microalbuminuria and non-insulin dependent diabetes: the candesartan and lisinopril microalbuminuria (CALM) study. BMJ 2000; 321(7274):1440–4.

114. Lewis EJ, Hunsicker LG, Clarke WR et al, Collaborative Study Group. Renoprotective effect of the angiotensin-receptor antagonist irbesartan in patients with nephropathy due to type 2 diabetes. New Engl J Med 2001; 345:851–60.

115. Brenner BM, Cooper ME, De Zeeuw D et al, RENAL study investigators. Effects of losartan on renal and cardiovascular outcomes in patients with type 2 diabetes and nephropathy. New Engl J Med 2001; 345:861–9.

116. Havranek EP, Thomas I, Smith WB et al. Dose-related beneficial long-term hemodynamic and clinical efficacy of irbesartan in heart failure. J Am Coll Cardiol 1999; 33(5):1174–81.

117. Elmfeldt D, George M, Hubner R, Olofsson B. Candesartan cilexetil, a new generation angiotensin II antagonist, provides dose dependent antihypertensive effect. J Hum Hypertens 1997; 11(Suppl 2):S49–53.

118. Guazzi M, Melzi G, Agostoni P. Comparison of changes in respiratory function and exercise oxygen uptake with losartan versus enalapril in congestive heart failure secondary to ischaemic or idiopathic dilated cardiomyopathy. Am J Cardiol 1997; 80:1572–6.

119. Warner JGJ Jr, Metzger DC, Kitzman DW, Wesley DJ, Little WC. Losartan improves exercise tolerance in patients with diastolic dysfunction and a hypertensive response to exercise. J Am Coll Cardiol 1999; 33:1567–72.

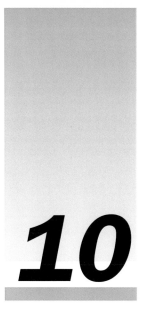

Cerebrovascular prevention by angiotensin II receptor antagonists

Massimo Volpe and Giuliano Tocci

10

Introduction

Cerebrovascular accidents represent one of the leading causes of morbidity and mortality worldwide.[1–4] According to the most recent reports, in the United States approximately 700 000 strokes occur each year, including 500 000 first attacks and 200 000 recurrent episodes.[2] A report of the World Health Organization (WHO) illustrates that in 1990 stroke accounted for 4.3 million lives each year, making it the third most common cause of death on the planet.[3] In the same report, the projection to year 2020 showed that stroke-related death is expected to rise to 7.7 millions.[3] In addition, stroke is the most frequent cause of disability, and about one-third of the individuals suffering a stroke are left with a major permanent disability.[3,4] Thus, the consequences of a stroke for patients, their families, and the healthcare systems are enormous, in view of the fact that more than 40% of stroke patients require active rehabilitation, with ongoing problems including physical handicap, cognitive dysfunction, and depression. For these reasons, the cost of stroke accounts for 3–4% of the total healthcare care costs in Western countries.[1]

Blood pressure elevation is the most common and powerful contributor to stroke.[5,6] In fact, hypertensive patients have a fourfold increased risk of stroke, as compared to the reference normotensive population.[5–8] Actually, starting at about 115 mmHg systolic blood pressure, cerebrovascular risk continuously and linearly increases by doubling for every 20 mmHg increment.[5] This implies that even within the traditional 'normotensive area' risk of stroke increases progressively with the elevation of blood pressure, and this relationship is enhanced by the concomitant presence of major risk factors or target organ damage.[9–11] In other words, three-quarters of all strokes occur among patients traditionally considered normotensive, and, even though high blood pressure can be identified as the most important modifiable risk factor for stroke, other factors may be implied in its pathogenesis.[12,13]

Hypertension is virtually implied in all mechanisms involved in the pathogenesis of different types of stroke.[14–18] Hypertension contributes to the *atherothrombotic* stroke type, the most frequent form of stroke, which accounts for more than 80% of the total.[19,20] It accelerates the atherosclerotic process that most frequently affects large precerebral arteries. High blood pressure is also the main factor involved in the production of adaptive changes (sclerosis, lypohyalinosis, microaneurysms) occurring in the wall of small parenchymal vessels of the brain in many hypertensive individuals, changes that lead to either *lacunar* ischemic stroke or to the *intraparenchymal hemorrhagic* type. Uncontrolled hypertension also promotes the formation and subsequent rupture of saccular aneurysms of middle-caliber intracranial arteries, causing the *subarachnoid hemorrhage* type of stroke. Even in the *cardioembolic* stroke type, hypertension plays a major role, particularly because it is involved in the mechanisms leading to atrial fibrillation, the first cause of embolic stroke.

The hypothesis that other mechanisms beyond high blood pressure are involved in the susceptibility to stroke in hypertension seems particularly plausible for the *atherothrombotic* or *ischemic* type of stroke, and it is supported by a large body of experimental and epidemiologic data.[21–23] For instance, the most common cause of death for a classical experimental model of stroke, the *stroke-prone* spontaneously hypertensive rat (SHRsp) is represented by *ischemic* stroke, despite the very high levels of blood pressure that these animals achieve.[24] On the other hand, the progressive improvement in the treatment management of hypertension in the last decades has been reflected by a dramatic reduction of *hemorrhagic* stroke, whereas *ischemic* stroke has been much less influenced by the blood pressure-lowering treatment, thus implying that other factors are involved.[25,26]

Randomized, controlled trials in hypertension have demonstrated that effective treatment of high blood pressure levels significantly reduces the incidence of all major cardiovascular events, mostly stroke, and several large meta-analyses have consistently demonstrated that effective blood pressure reduction lowers the incidence of stroke by about 40%.[27–31] In hypertensive patients with additional cardiovascular risk factors or clinical conditions such as diabetes, target organ damage, or associated clinical conditions, even small decreases in blood pressure levels are associated with large reductions in cerebrovascular risk.[12,13] Also epidemiologic surveys suggest that a less effective control of blood pressure is associated with a higher incidence of stroke in different countries.[5–8]

The benefits of blood pressure reductions, however, are not strictly proportional to stroke incidence.[12,13] Thus, it has been suggested that the different classes of antihypertensive drugs may have specific properties for organ protection and cerebrovascular accident prevention.[27–31] Beta-blockers (BBs), and (in general) more sympatholytic agents, may recognize an important additional property in their ability to block the sympathoadrenergic drive to heart and vessels, beyond the blood pressure-lowering effect.[32–33] Similarly, calcium channel blockers (CCBs) are thought to interfere with the atherosclerotic process besides the well-known blood pressure-lowering effects, and it has been often concluded that their properties may be particularly beneficial in terms of stroke prevention.[31] Finally, blocking the renin–angiotensin system (RAS) with angiotensin converting enzyme (ACE) inhibitors has been postulated as an effective strategy of reducing the risk of stroke, especially, in hypertensive patients, in view of the detrimental influence of angiotensin II on vascular structure and function.[25–28] However, the results of large meta-analyses do not support any specific advantages of one class over another in terms of stroke prevention in hypertension.[34–36] For these reasons, the prevailing current concept is that tight control of blood pressure levels can effectively reduce stroke-related morbidity and mortality, and there is no available proof that specific pleiotropic properties of these antihypertensive classes may provide additional stroke protection.

More recently, the availability of the results of large outcome studies with angiotensin II receptor antagonists or blockers (ARBs) in hypertension has generated new interest towards the possibility that other mechanisms, and particularly those related to the activity of the angiotensin II, participate in the etiopathogenesis of stroke in hypertension.[25–28] This chapter briefly reviews the recent clinical studies with ACE inhibitors and ARBs, with particular emphasis on stroke prevention in hypertension.

RAS and cerebrovascular protection

The possibility that angiotensin II is involved in the development of cerebrovascular diseases and stroke has long been investigated. Pioneering work by Laragh and co-workers in the early 1970s, initially described the vasculotoxic effects of angiotensin II and the development of stroke in experimental models.[37] Subsequently, the same group reported a higher stroke incidence in hypertensive patients with elevated levels of plasma renin activity.[38] Finally, studies by Volpe et al showed that in SHRsp ischemic stroke was strictly related to the inability to properly suppress renin activity in the presence of a high-salt Japanese-style diet.[39–41] Also in patients with a family history of stroke, an impaired regulation of the RAS has been reported.[42]

The availability of drugs selectively blocking angiotensin II receptors has recently prompted new, exciting research on the putative role of angiotensin II in the brain.[43–45] Two major receptor subtypes modulate the activity of angiotensin II in the adult: the AT_1 and the AT_2 receptors.[46] Of the two, AT_1 predominates and mediates all the classic physiologic effects of angiotensin II, including vasoconstriction, sodium and water retention, and release of aldosterone. It has also become clear that the AT_1 receptors mediate the pathophysiologic effects of angiotensin II, such as cell proliferation and growth, oxidative and inflammatory process, cardiac hypertrophy and dysfunction, atrial fibrillation, and endothelial dysfunction.[46] The AT_2 receptors, which appear to be mostly expressed in settings of injury or disease, mediate effects that are generally opposite to those of AT_1, such as vasorelaxation, growth inhibition, cell differentiation, and apoptosis.[46] In particular, the AT_2 receptors exert an important role in cellular differentiation in the brain, as discussed elsewhere in this book. Several experimental studies have suggested a neuroprotective action of the AT_2 receptors.[47–49] For instance, the neurologic deficit in rats due to ischemia is lessened by chronic pretreatment with losartan, but not by pretreatment with the AT_2 antagonist PD123177.[47] Combination of the two treatments abolishes the protective effects of losartan, indicating that, at least in part, the protective effects are mediated by selective stimulation of the AT_2 receptors. These and other observations (which are discussed more extensively in another chapter) indicate that drugs inhibiting the RAS at different levels may generate different effects on cerebral parenchyma and vasculature, and may contribute to explaining the different influence on cerebrovascular outcomes of ACE inhibitors and ARBs.

The complex organization of the RAS strictly interacts with other important biologic pathways, such as the kallikrein–kinin cascade and the nitric oxide–cyclic GMP system. Therefore, the different pharmacologic interventions that interact with the RAS (ACE inhibitors, ARBs, renin inhibitors) may prompt different outcomes in the cerebral circulation, as shown in Figure 10.1, and cannot be considered automatically interchangeable. Further investigations will clarify this issue.

Clinical trials with ACE inhibitors or ARBs and stroke

Clinical evidence supporting the cerebrovascular protective activity of RAS blocking agents has been provided by studies that show a reduced incidence of strokes with pharmacologic agents that counteract this system.[50–66] In this regard, suggestive data have been derived from the results of the Perindopril pROtection aGainst REcurrent Stroke Study (PROGRESS), which enrolled 6105 patients with a history of stroke within the previous 5 years, around half of whom were hypertensives (systolic blood pressure of 160 mmHg or diastolic blood pressure of 90 mmHg).[50] Patients were randomized to once-daily perindopril 4 mg or placebo, and those who had no contraindication for diuretics also received indapamide 2.5 mg. Although the reduction in systolic blood pressure with perindopril monotherapy was around 5 mmHg, compared with placebo, there was no significant reduction in the risk of recurrent stroke compared with placebo. In those patients who received combination therapy with perindopril and indapamide, there was a highly significant 40% reduction in the risk of stroke ($p < 0.01$) in the presence of a further significant lowering of systolic blood pressure levels (around 12 mmHg).[50]

In the Heart Outcomes Prevention Evaluation (HOPE) study a total of 9297 patients at high risk, 55 years of age or older, with evidence of vascular disease or diabetes mellitus or one

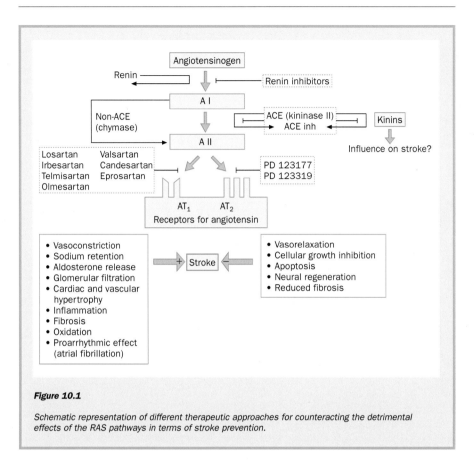

Figure 10.1

Schematic representation of different therapeutic approaches for counteracting the detrimental effects of the RAS pathways in terms of stroke prevention.

additive cardiovascular risk factor, were randomly assigned to receive ramipril (10 mg once daily orally) or matching placebo for a mean of 5 years of follow-up.[21] The primary outcome was a composite of myocardial infarction, stroke, or death from cardiovascular causes. Treatment with ramipril significantly reduced the rates of stroke (3.4% vs 4.9%; $p < 0.001$) in comparison with the treatment with placebo.[21] This benefit was attributed by the authors to factors that are considered as independent from the blood pressure reduction. However, a reduction of about 3 mmHg was indeed observed in the ACE inhibitor-treated group rather than in the placebo-treated group, and such a reduction can be considered meaningful in high-risk individuals. Also in this study, however, the more favorable influence of the antihypertensive strategy, including the ACE inhibitors, was associated with a larger and significant blood pressure reduction. Thus, a key role of the antihypertensive effect cannot be excluded.

More recently, the publication of the results of the Anglo–Scandinavian Cardiac Outcomes Trial – Blood Pressure Lowering Arm (ASCOT-BPLA) study has highlighted that the benefits of a CCB-based strategy with the addition of an ACE inhibitor, if necessary, in the prevention of stroke overrides those achieved with the traditional antihypertensive agents, based on the combination therapy between a BB and thiazide diuretic.[51,52] Although the study, which was originally powered for an estimated 1150 primary end points, was stopped prematurely when only 903 primary end points had occurred, the amlodipine–perindopril regimen was consistently better than the comparator regimen with atenolol–thiazide diuretic in terms of fatal and non-fatal stroke (reduction of 23%; $p = 0.003$).

In contrast to this evidence, which may be interpreted as favorable to the ACE inhibitor-based regimen, stand the results of the Antihypertensive and Lipid-Lowering treatment to prevent Heart Attack Trial (ALLHAT), which was designed to determine whether treatment with a CCB or an ACE inhibitor lowered the incidence of coronary heart disease or other cardiovascular disease events, including stroke, in comparison to the treatment with a diuretic.[53] A total of 33 357 subjects, aged 55 years old or older, with a history of hypertension and at least one other vascular risk factor, were randomly assigned to receive chlorthalidone 12.5–25 mg/day ($n = 15 255$); amlodipine 2.5–10 mg/day ($n = 9048$); or lisinopril 10–40 mg/day ($n = 9054$), and were followed-up for 4–8 years. In this study, the chlorthalidone-based regimen lowered blood pressure more than ACE inhibitors throughout the 10-year follow-up period. Focusing on the incidence of stroke, while the relative risk was non-significant comparing amlodipine with chlorthalidone (0.93; CI = 0.82–1.06), chlorthalidone proved superior to lisinopril (RR = 1.15; 95% CI = 1.02–1.30), particularly in black patients, in agreement with multiple reports of poorer blood pressure response to ACE inhibitors in this racial group of patients.[53]

Also the results of the Second Australian National Blood Pressure Study Group (ANBP2) do not fully support a superiority of ACE inhibitors over conventional therapy with regard to stroke incidence.[54] This study was a prospective, randomized, open-label study, which considered the total number of cardiovascular events, including stroke, in a population of 6083 subjects, aged 65 to 84 years old, with a history of hypertension. In the presence of comparable blood pressure reductions, the incidence of stroke was similar in two treatment groups (112 vs 107; RR = 1.02 (0.78–1.33); $p = 0.91$).[54] These two large trials seem to document that when ACE inhibitors do not induce a larger blood pressure response, the additional benefit in terms of stroke reduction is not present. As shown in Table 10.1, altogether the beneficial effects of ACE inhibitors on stroke in hypertension trials seem to be largely linked to the blood pressure-lowering effect. In particular, the studies showing a benefit with ACE inhibitors on stroke incidence in hypertension were systematically linked to the significant blood pressure-lowering effect of these drugs. Among the available vast meta-analyses, the Blood Pressure Lowering Treatment Trialists' Collaboration has undertaken a retrospective assessment of comparative clinical trials, showing that ACE inhibitor-based and CCB-based regimens reduce the risk of stroke as compared with placebo (by 28% (95% CI = 19–36); and 38% (95% CI = 18–53), respectively).[27,28] When the efficacy of the ACE inhibitor regimen on stroke prevention was tested against conventional therapy, the ACE inhibitor-based therapy was marginally less effective at preventing total (fatal and non-fatal) stroke. It is important to point out again that in the two main studies showing

Table 10.1
Stroke incidence in recent hypertension trials with ACE inhibitors or ARBs.

Trial	Year	Drug	Comparator	BP difference (mmHg)	Population (n)	Number of stroke (drug/comparator)	Stroke reduction	p value
ACE inhibitor								
STOP2	1999	ACE inh	BBs/HCTZ	+1.0/0.0*	6.614	(nr)	0.90 (0.74–1.08)	0.24
CAPPP	1999	Captopril	BBs/HCTZ	(nr)*	10.985	224/174	1.43 (1.12–1.82)	0.004
UKPDS	1998	Captopril	Atenolol	1/2*	1.148	21/17	1.12 (0.59–2.12)	0.74
HOPE	2000	Ramipril	Placebo	3/1[†]	9.297	156/226	0.68 (0.56–0.84)	<0.001
PROGRESS	2001	Perindopril	Placebo	9/4[†]	6.105	307/420	0.72 (0.62–0.83)	<0.001
ANBP2	2003	ACE inh	Diuretics	0/0*	6.083	112/107	1.02 (0.78–1.33)	0.91
ALLHAT-BPLA	2002	Lisinopril	Chlorthalidone	+2.0[†]	33.357	457/675	1.15 (1.02–1.30)	0.02
ASCOTT-BPLA	2005	Amlodipine/perindopril	Atenolol/HCTZ	3/2[†]	19.257	307/422	0.77 (0.66–0.89)	0.0003
ARBs								
LIFE	2002	Losartan	Atenolol	1.1/0.2*	9193	232/309	0.75 (0.63–0.89)	<0.001
SCOPE	2003	Candesartan	Placebo	3/1[†]	4964	89/115	0.76 (0.58–1.1)	0.056
VALUE	2004	Valsartan	Amlodipine	+2.2/+1.6[†]	15.245	322/281	1.15 (0.98–1.35)	0.08
MOSES	2005	Eprosartan	Nitrendipine	1.5/0.6*	1405	206/255	0.75 (0.58–0.97)	0.026

In the UKPDS, HOPE, ALLHAT, LIFE, SCOPE, and VALUE studies, the number of events includes fatal and non-fatal stroke; in the PROGRESS study, the number of events includes fatal or disabling and non-fatal stroke; in the CAPPP study, the number of events includes fatal and non-fatal stroke and transient ischemic attack; in the MOSES study, the number of events includes fatal and non-fatal stroke and recurrent events. ACE inh, ACE inhibitors; CCBs, calcium channel blockers; BBs, β-blockers; *not significant; *p < 0.05; [†]p < 0.001.

greater reductions in terms of stroke prevention with ACE inhibitor-based treatment compared with placebo, the PROGRESS trial[50] and the HOPE study,[21] these benefits were observed in the presence of significantly greater blood pressure reductions in the active treatment groups than in placebo groups. As previously discussed, these differences in blood pressure are more than sufficient to account for the cardiovascular benefits observed in these two trials. Moreover, when ACE inhibition has been compared 'head-to-head' with other blood pressure-lowering drugs, such as in the ALLHAT trial,[53] in the ANBP2,[54] in the Swedish Trial in Old Patients with Hypertension-2 (STOP2),[55] and in the CAptopril Prevention Project (CAPPP),[56] there is no suggestion from any of these trials of superior stroke prevention by ACE inhibition vs other antihypertensive therapies.

In contrast to what is observed with ACE inhibitors, a beneficial effect on stroke with ARBs has been observed also in the presence of comparable blood pressure reductions, as illustrated in Table 10.1. This interpretation is consistently validated by several recent meta-analyses, thus supporting the concept that ARBs provide protective effects in terms of stroke incidence reduction beyond blood pressure control. On average, in the Blood Pressure Lowering Treatment Trialists' Collaboration meta-analysis,[27,28] the risk of stroke was significantly reduced with ARB-based regimens compared with other active treatment, including BBs, CCBs, and diuretics (21% (95% CI = 10–31)), as shown in Figure 10.2.

In this regard, very strong and convincing evidence that ARBs have favorable effects on the risk of stroke that go beyond blood pressure reductions can be derived from the Losartan Intervention For Endpoint reduction (LIFE) study, which recruited more than 9000 patients

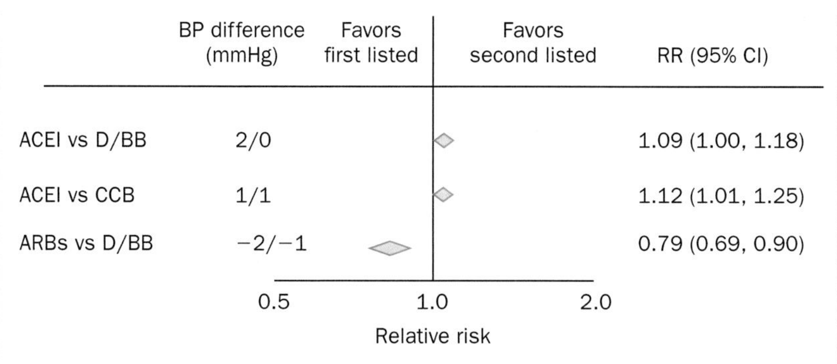

	BP difference (mmHg)	Favors first listed	Favors second listed	RR (95% CI)
ACEI vs D/BB	2/0	◇		1.09 (1.00, 1.18)
ACEI vs CCB	1/1	◇		1.12 (1.01, 1.25)
ARBs vs D/BB	−2/−1	◇		0.79 (0.69, 0.90)
	0.5	1.0	2.0	
		Relative risk		

Figure 10.2

Comparison between angiotensin converting enzyme inhibitors (ACEI), calcium channel blockers (CCBs), β-blockers (BBs), angiotensin II receptor blockers (ARBs) and diuretics (D) in terms of reduction of stroke. BP, blood pressure; CI, confidence interval; RR, relative risk. From Turnbull.[28]

with hypertension and left ventricular hypertrophy.[57] A treatment regimen based on the ARB losartan (about 90% of patients received combination therapy) produced quite comparable blood pressure reductions to the treatment regimen based on the BB atenolol, as illustrated in Figure 10.3. However, the losartan-based regimen significantly reduced the risk of the primary composite end point (cardiovascular death, stroke, and myocardial infarction) compared with the atenolol-based regimen. In particular, losartan significantly reduced the incidence of fatal and non-fatal stroke compared with atenolol in hypertensive patients with left ventricular hypertrophy. Similar additional benefits on stroke, in the presence of comparable effects on blood pressure, were observed in the patients treated with losartan vs those treated with atenolol in the cohorts of patients with diabetes mellitus[58] and patients with isolated systolic hypertension.[59] Further substudies from LIFE have demonstrated that losartan effectively reduced left ventricular hypertrophy and left atrial dimensions more than atenolol,[60,61] and was more effective in preventing the new onset of atrial fibrillation in patients in sinus rhythm (more than 8000 patients)[60] or maintaining sinus rhythm after an episode of atrial fibrillation.[61] These effects of losartan may contribute to reducing the risk of ischemic stroke.

The Study on COgnition and Prognosis in the Elderly (SCOPE), which recruited elderly patients with predominantly systolic hypertension, demonstrated the ability of the ARB candesartan to produce a statistically significant 28% reduction in the incidence of non-fatal stroke and a non-significant 24% reduction in total stroke compared with placebo (which was indeed mostly active treatment), after a 4-year follow-up.[62] These results, however, could be partly explained by a difference in blood pressure between the two arms (amounting in this case to 3.2/1.6 mmHg in favor of candesartan).

The Valsartan Antihypertensive Long-term Use Evaluation (VALUE) trial was a prospective, multinational, double-blind, randomized, active-controlled, parallel group study which aimed at comparing for the 'same level of achieved blood pressure' the long-term effects of antihypertensive therapy on the incidence of cardiovascular morbidity and mortality.[63,64] For this purpose, 15 245 patients were randomly assigned to a valsartan-based regimen (7649 patients) or to an amlodipine-based regimen (7596 patients). Patients enrolled were 50 years old or older, with a history of hypertension and predefined combinations of cardiovascular risk factors (including age older than 50 years old, male sex, diabetes mellitus, current smoking, high total cholesterol, left ventricular hypertrophy, proteinuria, and raised serum creatinine) or cardiovascular diseases (including coronary disease, cerebrovascular disease, or peripheral arterial occlusive disease). Mean follow-up time was 4.2 years. The primary end point was time to first cardiac event, while fatal and non-fatal stroke was considered as a secondary end point, together with myocardial infarction and heart failure. Unfortunately, for the objective interpretation of the study, the amlodipine-based regimen caused a greater blood pressure reduction than valsartan throughout the study, and especially during the first 6 months of the follow-up, during which the highest frequency of cardiovascular events, including stroke, was recorded. Fatal and non-fatal stroke was slightly less in the amlodipine group, since it occurred in 4.2% of patients

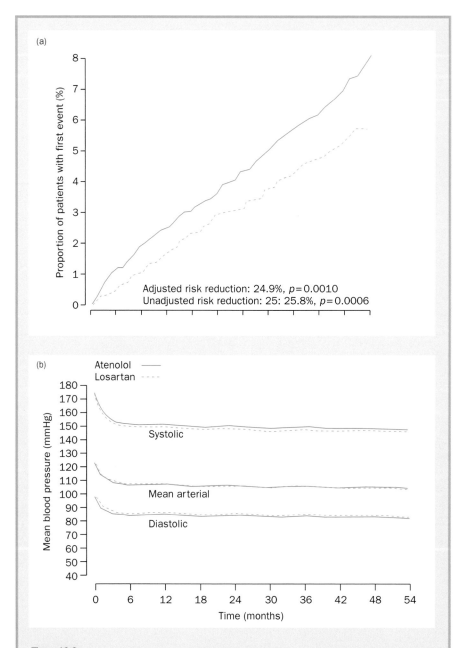

Figure 10.3

(a) Kaplan-Meier curves for the incidence of the (fatal and non-fatal) stroke end point in the LIFE trial
(b) Mean blood pressure values during follow-up.

in the valsartan group and in 3.7% of patients in the amlodipine group (hazard ratio = 1.15; 95% CI = 0.98–1.35; p = 0.08).[63,64]

Finally, the MOrbidity and mortality after Stroke – Eprosartan compared with nitrendipine for Secondary prevention (MOSES) study enrolled a total of 1405 hypertensives with a history of cerebrovascular events, randomized to an antihypertensive regimen based on either the ARB eprosartan or the CCB nitrendipine 10 mg.[65] Inclusion criteria were hypertension requiring pharmacologic treatment and a history of cerebrovascular events (transient ischemic attack, focal neurologic deficit attributable to ischemia resolving within 24 hours, ischemic stroke, and cerebral hemorrhage), documented by either cranial computed tomography or magnetic resonance scan (within the past 24 months before inclusion). Primary end point was the composite of all-cause mortality and the number of cardiovascular and cerebrovascular events, including all recurrent events. Cerebral complications were defined as intracerebral hemorrhage, recurrence of stroke, or transient ischemic attack or prolonged reversible ischemic neurologic deficit. Cardiovascular complications were defined as any cardiovascular event (including myocardial infarction and new cardiac failure). Secondary end points were all single components of the combined primary end point. Further prespecified secondary end points were assessment of the patient's functional capacity and mental function. The blood pressure reduction was comparable in the two study groups without any significant detectable difference throughout the study period. Actually, at the end of the study, mean office blood pressure was 137.5/80.8 mmHg with the eprosartan-based regimens and 136.0/80.2 mmHg with the nitrendipine-based regimens.[65] As shown in Figure 10.4, despite the similar blood pressure control, the eprosartan-based regimen lowered primary end points significantly more than the nitrendipine group. A total of 461 (fatal and non-fatal, including recurrences of stroke) events occurred: 206 (13.3%) in the eprosartan group and 255 (16.7%) in the nitrendipine (p = 0.014).[65] Considering cerebrovascular events, a total of 236 fatal and non-fatal events occurred, 102 (43.2%) in the eprosartan group and 134 (56.8%) in the nitrendipine group (p = 0.026).[65]

Together with the previous studies analyzing stroke incidence with ARBs and other various comparators, the MOSES study reinforces the hypothesis that ARBs may exert cerebrovascular protection beyond the blood pressure-lowering effect. Whether this action is linked to inhibition of RAS or the specific interaction of ARBs with the angiotensin II receptor network is unclear at this time. The results of the ONTARGET/TRASCEND study, a large trial comparing the AT_1 receptor blocker telmisartan with the ACE inhibitor ramipril and the combination of the two in high-risk individuals may provide further support to this important aspect in the chemical management of patients at high-risk. In fact,[66] stroke incidence will be an interesting end point and the findings of this study may be helpful to further clarify the items discussed above.

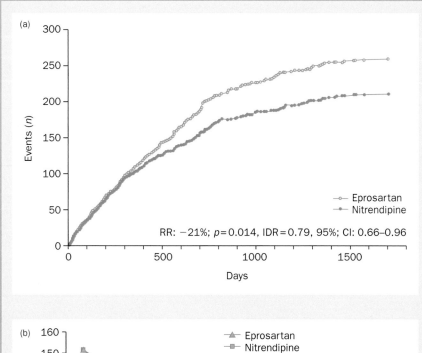

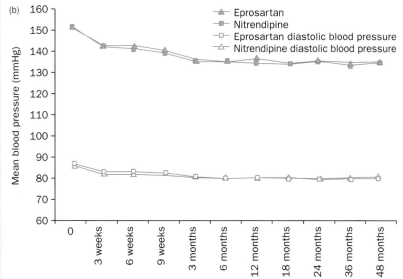

Figure 10.4

(a) Kaplan–Meier curves for the incidence of the primary end point in the MOSES trial. (b) Mean blood pressure values during follow-up. From Schrader et al.[65]

Summary

Stroke represents the most devastating cardiovascular disease in Western countries, occurring each year in 30.9 million individuals worldwide and being responsible for approximately 4 million deaths. High blood pressure is the most relevant, modifiable risk factor for developing stroke. In addition, angiotensin II is an important driving pathophysiological mechanism in stroke, and several levels of evidence indicate that selective blockade of angiotensin II at receptor levels and possibly the concomitant binding of angiotensin II to the AT_2 receptors may effectively antagonize the key mechanisms involved in the pathogenesis of stroke.

In hypertensive patients, especially those with additional cardiovascular risk factors or clinical settings such as diabetes, target organ damage, or associated clinical conditions, even small decreases in blood pressure levels are associated with large reductions in incidence of cerebrovascular events. The benefits of blood pressure reductions, however, are not strictly proportional to stroke incidence. Thus, it has been suggested that the different classes of antihypertensive drugs may have specific properties for organ protection and cerebrovascular accident prevention. The results of the available clinical trials document an efficacy of ARBs on stroke prevention on top of the antihypertensive effect. In particular, the hypothesis of a greater cerebrovascular protection by AT_1 type angiotensin II receptor blockers is an attractive perspective that deserves further investigations.

References

1. Olesen J, Leonardi M. The burden of brain diseases in Europe. Eur J Neurol 2003; 10(5):471–7.
2. Eyre H, Kahn R, Robertson RM et al, on behalf of the American Cancer Society, American Diabetes Association and American Heart Association. Preventing cancer, cardiovascular disease, and diabetes: a common agenda for the American Cancer Society, the American Diabetes Association, and the American Heart Association. Stroke 2004; 35(8):1999–2010.
3. Stroke – 1989. Recommendations on stroke prevention, diagnosis, and therapy. Report of the WHO Task Force on Stroke and other Cerebrovascular Disorders. Stroke 1989; 20(10):1407–31.
4. Adams RJ, Chimowitz MI, Alpert JS et al. Coronary risk evaluation in patients with transient ischemic attack and ischemic stroke: a scientific statement for healthcare professionals from the Stroke Council and the Council on Clinical Cardiology of the American Heart Association/American Stroke Association. Stroke 2003; 34:2310–22.
5. MacMahon S, Peto R, Cutler J et al. Blood pressure, stroke, and coronary heart disease. Part 1, Prolonged differences in blood pressure: prospective observational studies corrected for the regression dilution bias. Lancet 1990; 335:765–74.
6. Collins R, Peto R, MacMahon S et al. Blood pressure, stroke, and coronary heart disease. Part 2, Short-term reductions in blood pressure: overview of randomised drug trials in their epidemiological context. Lancet 1990; 335:827–39.
7. Vasan RS, Larson MG, Leip EP et al. Impact of high-normal blood pressure on the risk of cardiovascular disease. New Engl J Med 2001; 345(18):1291–7.
8. Lewington S, Clarke R, Qizilbash N et al, for the Prospective Studies Collaboration. Age-specific relevance of usual blood pressure to vascular mortality: a meta-analysis of individual data for one million adults in 61 prospective studies. Lancet 2002; 360:1903–13.
9. Anderson KM, Odell PM, Wilson PW, Kannel WB. Cardiovascular disease risk profile. Am Heart J 1991; 121:293–8.

10. Andersson OK, Almgren T, Persson B et al. Survival in treated hypertension: follow up study after two decades. BMJ 1998; 317:167–71.

11. Almgren T, Persson B, Wilhelmson L et al. Stroke and coronary heart disease in treated hypertension – a prospective cohort study ove three decades. J Intern Med 2005; 257(6):496–502.

12. Alderman MH, Furberg CD, Kostis JB et al. Hypertension guidelines: criteria that might make them more clinically useful. Am J Hypertens 2002; 15(10 Pt 1):917–23.

13. Volpe M, Alderman MH, Furberg CD et al. Beyond hypertension toward guidelines for cardiovascular risk reduction. Am J Hypertens 2004; 17(11 Pt 1):1068–74.

14. Neaton JD, Wentworth D. Serum cholesterol, blood pressure, cigarette smoking and death from coronary heart disease. Overall findings and differences by age for 316,099 white men. Multiple Risk Factor Intervention Trial (MRFIT) Research Group. Arch Intern Med 1992; 152:56–64.

15. Kjeldsen SE, Julius S, Hedner T, Hansson L. Stroke is more common than myocardial infarction in hypertension: analysis based on 11 major randomized intervention trials. Blood Press 2001; 10:190–2.

16. SHEP Cooperative Research Group. Prevention of stroke by antihypertensive drug treatment in older persons with isolated systolic hypertension. Final results of the Systolic Hypertension in the Elderly Program (SHEP). JAMA 1991; 265:3255–64.

17. Staessen JA, Fagard R, Thijs L et al, for the Systolic Hypertension in Europe (Syst-Eur) Trial Investigators. Randomised double-blind comparison of placebo and active treatment for older patients with isolated systolic hypertension. Lancet 1997; 350:757–64.

18. Fagard RH, Staessen JA, Thijs L et al. Response to antihypertensive therapy in older patients with sustained and nonsustained systolic hypertension. Systolic Hypertension in Europe (Syst-Eur) Trial Investigators. Circulation 2000; 102(10):1139–44.

19. Mancia G. Prevention and treatment of stroke in patients with hypertension. Clin Ther 2004; 26(5):631–48.

20. Mancia G, Ambrosioni E, Rosei EA et al, for the ForLife study group. Blood pressure control and risk of stroke in untreated and treated hypertensive patients screened from clinical practice: results of the ForLife study. J Hypertens 2005; 23(8):1575–81.

21. Yusuf S, Sleight P, Dagenais G et al, for the Heart Outcomes Prevention Evaluation (HOPE) Study Group. Effects of angiotensin-converting enzyme inhibitor, ramipril, on cardiovascular events in high-risk patients. N Engl J Med 2000; 342:145–53.

22. Hansson L, Zanchetti A, Carruthers SG et al, for the HOT Study Group. Effects of intensive blood-pressure lowering and low-dose aspirin in patients with hypertension: principal results of the Hypertension Optimal Treatment (HOT) randomised trial. Lancet 1998; 351:1755–62.

23. Zanchetti A, Hansson L, Dahlöf B et al, for the HOT Study Group. Effects of individual risk factors on the incidence of cardiovascular events in the treated hypertensive patients of the Hypertension Optimal Treatment (HOT) Study. J Hypertens 2001; 19:1149–59.

24. Cosentino F, Savoia C, De Paolis P et al. Angiotensin II type 2 receptors contribute to vascular responses in spontaneously hypertensive rats treated with angiotensin II type 1 receptor antagonists. Am J Hypertens 2005; 18(4 Pt 1):493–9.

25. Volpe M, Ruilope LM, McInnes GT, Waeber B, Weber MA. Angiotensin-II receptor blockers: benefits beyond blood pressure reduction? J Hum Hypertens 2005; 19; 331–9.

26. Ruilope LM, Rosei EA, Bakris GL et al. Angiotensin receptor blockers: therapeutic targets and cardiovascular protection. Blood Press 2005; 14(4):196–209.

27. Neal B, MacMahon S, Chapman N. Effects of ACE inhibitors, calcium antagonists, and other blood-pressure-lowering drugs: results of prospectively designed overviews of randomized trials. Blood Pressure Lowering Treatment Trialists Collaboration. Lancet 2000; 356:1955–64.

28. Turnbull F, Blood Pressure Lowering Treatment Trialists' Collaboration. Effects of different blood-pressure-lowering regimens on major cardiovascular events: results of prospectively-designed overviews of randomised trials. Lancet 2003; 362:1527–35.

29. Pahor M, Psaty BM, Alderman MH et al. Health outcomes associated with calcium antagonists compared with other first-line antihypertensive therapies: a meta-analysis of randomised controlled trials. Lancet 2000; 356:1949–54.

30. Angeli F, Verdecchia P, Reboldi GP et al. Calcium channel blockade to prevent stroke in hypertension: a meta-analysis of 13 studies with 130,793 subjects. Am J Hypertens 2004; 17:817–22.

31. Verdecchia P, Reboldi G, Angeli F et al. Angiotensin-converting enzyme inhibitors and calcium channel blockers for coronary heart disease and stroke prevention. Hypertension 2005; 46:386–92.

32. Lindholm LH, Carlberg B, Samuelsson O. Should beta blockers remain first choice in the treatment of primary hypertension? A meta-analysis. Lancet 2005; 366(9496):1545–53.

33. Messerli MH. Calcium antagonists and beta-blockers: impact on cardiovascular and cerebrovascular events. Clin Cornerstone 2004; 6(4):18–27.

34. 2003 World Health Organization (WHO)/International Society of Hypertension (ISH) statement on management of hypertension. J Hypertens 2003; 21:1983–92.

35. Chobanian A, Bakris G, Black H et al. The Seventh Report of the Joint National Committee on Prevention, Detection, Evaluation, and Treatment of High Blood Pressure: The JNC 7 Report. JAMA 2003; 289:2560–71.

36. 2003 European Society of Hypertension (ESH)/European Society of Cardiology (ESC) guidelines for the management of arterial hypertension. J Hypertension 2003; 21:1011–53.

37. Devereux RB, Pickering TG, Cody RJ, Laragh JH. Relation of renin–angiotensin system activity to left ventricular hypertrophy and function in experimental and human hypertension. J Clin Hypertens 1987; 3(1):87–103.

38. Volpe M, Camargo MJ, Mueller FB et al. Relation of plasma renin to end organ damage and to protection of K⁺ feeding in stroke-prone hypertensive rats. Hypertension 1990; 15(3):318–26.

39. Volpe M, Rubattu S, Ganten D et al. Dietary salt excess unmasks blunted aldosterone suppression and sodium retention in the stroke-prone phenotype of the spontaneously hypertensive rat. J Hypertens 1993; 11(8):793–8.

40. Volpe M, Iaccarino G, Vecchione C et al. Association and cosegregation of stroke with impaired endothelium-dependent vasorelaxation in stroke prone, spontaneously hypertensive rats. J Clin Invest 1996; 98(2):256–61.

41. Rubattu S, Lee-Kirsch MA, DePaolis P et al. Altered structure, regulation, and function of the gene encoding the atrial natriuretic peptide in the stroke-prone spontaneously hypertensive rat. Circ Res 1999; 85(10):900–5.

42. Volpe M, Lembo G, De Luca N et al. Abnormal hormonal and renal responses to saline load in hypertensive patients with parental history of cardiovascular accidents. Circulation 1991; 84(1):92–100.

43. Pu Q, Schiffrin EL. Effect of ACE/NEP inhibition on cardiac and vascular collagen in stroke-prone spontaneously hypertensive rats. Am J Hypertens 2001; 14(10):1067–72.

44. Kim S, Zhan Y, Izumi Y et al. In vivo activation of rat aortic platelet-derived growth factor and epidermal growth factor receptors by angiotensin II and hypertension. Arterioscler Thromb Vasc Biol 2000; 20(12):2539–45.

45. Brosnan MJ, Hamilton CA, Graham D et al. Irbesartan lowers superoxide levels and increases nitric oxide bioavailability in blood vessels from spontaneously hypertensive stroke-prone rats. J Hypertens 2002; 20(2):281–6.

46. Volpe M, Musumeci B, De Paolis P et al. Angiotensin II AT2 receptor subtype: an uprising frontier in cardiovascular disease? J Hypertens 2003; 21(8):1429–43.

47. Chrysant SG. Stroke prevention with losartan in the context of other antihypertensive drugs. Drugs Today 2004; 40(9):791–801.

48. Zimmerman MC, Lazartigues E, Sharma RV, Davisson RL. Hypertension caused by angiotensin II infusion involves increased superoxide production in the central nervous system. Circ Res 2004; 95(2):210–16.

49. Oku N, Kitagawa K, Imaizumi M et al. Hemodynamic influences of losartan on the brain in hypertensive patients. Hypertens Res 2005; 28(1):43–9.

50. The Perindopril pROtection aGainst REcurrent Stroke Study (PROGRESS) Collaborative Group. Randomized trial of perindopril-based blood-pressure-lowering regimen among 6105 individuals with previous stroke or transient ischaemic attack. Lancet 2001; 358:1033–41.

51. Dahlof B, Sever PS, Poulter NR et al, for the ASCOT Investigators. Prevention of cardiovascular events with an antihypertensive regimen of amlodipine adding perindopril as required versus atenolol adding bendroflumethiazide as required, in the Anglo-Scandinavian Cardiac Outcomes Trial-Blood

Pressure Lowering Arm (ASCOT-BPLA): a multicentre randomised controlled trial. Lancet 2005; 366(9489):895–906.

52. Poulter NR, Wedel H, Dahlof B et al, for the ASCOT Investigators. Role of blood pressure and other variables in the differential cardiovascular event rates noted in the Anglo-Scandinavian Cardiac Outcomes Trial–Blood Pressure Lowering Arm (ASCOT-BPLA). Lancet 2005; 366(9489):907–13.

53. ALLHAT Officers and Coordinators for the ALLHAT Collaborative Research Group. The Antihypertensive and Lipid-Lowering Treatment to Prevent Heart Attack Trial. Major outcomes in high-risk hypertensive patients randomized to angiotensin-converting enzyme inhibitor or calcium channel blocker vs diuretic: The Antihypertensive and Lipid-Lowering Treatment to Prevent Heart Attack Trial (ALLHAT). JAMA 2002; 288:2981–97.

54. Wing L, Reid C, Ryan P, Beilin L et al, for the Second Australian National Blood Pressure Study Group (ANBP2). A comparison of outcomes with angiotensin-converting-enzyme inhibitors and diuretics for hypertension in the elderly. N Engl J Med 2003; 348(7):583–92.

55. Hansson L, Lindholm LH, Ekbom T et al. Randomised trial of old and new antihypertensive drugs on cardiovascular mortality and morbidity in elderly patients with hypertension: the Swedish Trial in Old Patients with Hypertension-2 (STOP-2). Lancet 1999; 354:1751–6.

56. Niklason A, Hedner T, Niskanen L, Lanke J et al, for the CAPPP Study Group. Development of diabetes is retarded by ACE inhibition in hypertensive patients. A subanalysis of the CAPtopril Prevention Project (CAPPP). J Hypertens 2004; 22(3):645–52.

57. Dahlof B, Devereux RB, Kjeldsen SE et al, for the LIFE Study Group. Cardiovascular morbidity and mortality in the Losartan Intervention For End-point reduction in hypertension (LIFE) study: a randomised trial against atenolol. Lancet 2002; 359:995–1003.

58. Lindholm LH, Ibsen H, Dahlöf B et al, for the LIFE study group. Cardiovascular morbidity and mortality in patients with diabetes in the Losartan Intervention For Endpoint reduction in hypertension (LIFE) study: a randomised trial against atenolol. Lancet 2002; 359:1004–10.

59. Kjeldsen SE, Dahlof B, Devereux RB et al, LIFE (Losartan Intervention For Endpoint reduction) Study Group. Effects of losartan on cardiovascular morbidity and mortality in patients with isolated systolic hypertension and left ventricular hypertrophy: a Losartan Intervention For Endpoint reduction in hypertension (LIFE) substudy. JAMA 2002; 288(12):1491–8.

60. Wachtell K, Hornestam B, Lehto M et al. Cardiovascular morbidity and mortality in hypertensive patients with a history of atrial fibrillation. The Losartan Intervention For Endpoint reduction in hypertension (LIFE) study. J Am Coll Cardiol 2005; 45(5):705–11.

61. Wachtell K, Lehto M, Gerdts E et al. Angiotensin II receptor blockade reduces new-onset atrial fibrillation and subsequent stroke compared to atenolol. The Losartan Intervention For Endpoint reduction in hypertension (LIFE) study. J Am Coll Cardiol 2005; 45(5):712–19.

62. Lithell H, Hansson L, Skoog I et al, for the SCOPE Study Group. The Study on COgnition and Prognosis in the Elderly (SCOPE); outcomes in patients not receiving add-on therapy after randomization. J Hypertens 2004; 22(8):1605–12.

63. Julius S, Kjeldsen SE, Weber M et al, for the VALUE trial group. Outcomes in hypertensive patients at high cardiovascular risk treated with regimens based on valsartan or amlodipine: the Valsartan Antihypertensive Long-term Use Evaluation (VALUE) randomised trial. Lancet 2004; 363(9426):2022–31.

64. Weber MA, Julius S, Kjeldsen SE et al. Blood pressure dependent and independent effects of antihypertensive treatment on clinical events in the Valsartan Antihypertensive Long-term Use Evaluation (VALUE) Trial. Lancet 2004; 363(9426):2049–51.

65. Schrader J, Luders S, Kulschewski A et al, for the MOrbidity and Mortality after Stroke, Eprosartan compared with nitrendipine for Secondary prevention (MOSES) Study Group. Principal results of a prospective randomized controlled study. Stroke 2005; 36(6):1218–26.

66. Teo K, Yusuf S, Sleight P et al, for the ONTARGET/TRANSCEND Investigators. Rationale, design, and baseline characteristics of 2 large, simple, randomized trials evaluating telmisartan, ramipril, and their combination in high-risk patients: the ONgoing Telmisartan Alone and in combination with Ramipril Global Endpoint Trial/Telmisartan Randomized Assessment Study in ACE intolerant subjects with cardiovascular Disease (ONTARGET/TRANSCEND) trials. Am Heart J 2004; 148(1):52–61.

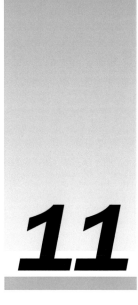

Past and ongoing trials with angiotensin II antagonists: data and perspectives regarding the treatment of hypertension

11

Sverre E Kjeldsen

Introduction

Clinical trials have examined whether angiotensin receptor blockers (ARBs) provide a greater reduction in the risk of cardiovascular end points and/or new-onset diabetes compared with older therapies such as diuretics, β-blockers, and calcium channel blockers in patients with hypertension.[1,2] This chapter reviews trial design and results of the completed Losartan Intervention For Endpoint reduction in hypertension (LIFE), Study on COgnition and Prognosis in the Elderly (SCOPE), MOrbidity and mortality after Stroke, Eprosartan compared with nitrendipine for Secondary prevention (MOSES), and Valsartan Antihypertensive Long-term Use Evaluation (VALUE) studies, and, briefly, the ONgoing Telmisartan Alone and in combination with Ramipril Global Endpoint Trial (ONTARGET), Telmisartan Randomized AssessmeNt Study in aCE iNtolerant subjects with cardiovascular Disease (TRANSCEND), Scandinavian Candesartan Acute Stroke Trial (SCAST), and Randomized Olmesartan And Diabetes MicroAlbuminuria Prevention Study (ROADMAP) studies.

LIFE

Design

The Losartan Intervention For Endpoint reduction in hypertension (LIFE) study was a double-blind, randomized study carried out on 9193 patients in seven countries. The aim was to study the effects of long-term treatment (≥4 years) with losartan- compared with atenolol-based therapy in patients with hypertension and electrocardiographic (ECG) evidence of left ventricular hypertrophy (LVH). The primary outcome was composite cardiovascular morbidity and mortality defined as myocardial infarction (MI), stroke, and cardiovascular mortality.[3] Prespecified analyses included analysis of patients with diabetes and isolated systolic hypertension (ISH) at baseline, development of new-onset diabetes, and ECG, echocardiographic, and microalbuminuria substudies.

Hypertension was documented following a 2-week, single-blind placebo period. Patients were eligible with sitting trough diastolic blood pressure (BP) of 95–115 mmHg and/or systolic BP of 160–200 mmHg, allowing for patients with ISH. ECG-LVH was defined as Cornell product ([RaVL + SV$_3$] × QRS duration) >2440 mm ms in men, with an added gender adjustment of 8 mm for women that was later reduced to 6 mm,[4] or Sokolow–Lyon voltage (SV$_1$ + RV$_5$ or V$_6$) >38 mm. Exclusion criteria included stroke or MI within 6 months.

Following randomization, patients received either losartan or atenolol 50 mg daily. If goal BP (140/90 mmHg) was not attained after 2 months, hydrochlorothiazide (HCTZ) 12 mg was added. After an additional 2 months, if goal BP was still not achieved, losartan or atenolol was doubled to 100 mg. Those still above target following an additional 2 months were to receive either an additional HCTZ 12.5 mg or other open-label antihypertensive agents, excluding angiotensin converting enzyme inhibitors (ACEIs), ARBs, or β-blockers. Titration to other open-label agents after this time was necessary only if BP was ≥165/95 mmHg.[3]

Analysis in this study was by intention-to-treat and the study was powered to detect a relative difference in the primary composite end point of 15% with 80% power and a two-sided significance level of 5%. Sample size was calculated so that with an absolute event rate over 5 years of 15% in the atenolol group and 12.75% in the losartan group, 1040 primary end points would be necessary. Background data to calculate a Framingham risk score[5] were obtained and used to adjust hazard ratios (HRs) associated with treatment.

Demographics, blood pressure control, and medications

Mean BP was 174/98 mmHg at randomization, reflecting elevated systolic hypertension in older patients (average age 66.9 years old). More patients satisfied the Cornell product than the Sokolow–Lyon voltage criteria for LVH, contributing to a mean voltage with the latter (30.0 ± 10.5 mm) that was actually lower than the entry criteria of 38 mm. Other important characteristics were elevated mean body mass index (BMI) of 28.0 kg/m^2 and 92% of patients who classified themselves ethnically as white (*n* = 533 black race).

BP was similarly controlled in the losartan and atenolol arms. Systolic BP at the end of follow-up or at the last visit before a primary event had fallen by 30.2 ± 18.5 mmHg in the losartan and by 29.1 ± 19.2 mmHg in the atenolol groups (*p* = 0.017). Diastolic BP had declined by

16.1 ± 10.1 and 16.8 ± 10.1 mmHg in the losartan and atenolol groups, respectively ($p = 0.37$). Mean arterial pressure was nearly identical, 102.2 and 102.4 mmHg, for the losartan and atenolol groups, respectively. The average dosages were losartan 82 mg and the atenolol 79 mg daily, and the majority of participants required HCTZ or another open-label antihypertensive.

Outcomes

The main finding in LIFE was that 11% of patients treated with losartan compared with 13% treated with atenolol experienced a primary end point, with an adjusted (for Framingham risk score) risk reduction (RR) of 13%, $p = 0.021$ (Table 11.1).[6] The most significant contributor to the composite end point was stroke, with rates of 10.8/1000 patient-years for losartan and 14.5/1000 patient-years for atenolol (25% RR, $p = 0.001$ adjusted). The atenolol group did not differ from the losartan group in the end points of MI and cardiovascular mortality.

New-onset diabetes was less frequent in the losartan group (25% RR, $p = 0.001$).[7] Other prespecified end points did not attain statistical significance (cardiovascular mortality, total mortality, hospitalization for heart failure, revascularization, MI, hospitalization for angina, and resuscitated cardiac arrest).

Substudies

The patients with ISH[8] represented an older portion of the LIFE study, whereas those patients in the group without clinically evident cardiovascular disease (no CVD) were younger.[9] Patients with diabetes[10] had an increased BMI and a higher Framingham risk score. Black patients, though a small portion of the overall LIFE cohort, comprised a greater percentage of patients within the diabetic subgroup. The sample sizes in the ISH and diabetic groups were smaller, decreasing the power to detect statistically significant results, than in the no CVD group.

The ISH and diabetic groups experienced a greater rate of outcomes than the overall LIFE and no CVD populations, underscoring the more serious nature of systolic hypertension and diabetes as a concomitant risk factor. Also, the LIFE study overall and subgroup analyses corroborate the finding that stroke is a more common outcome than MI in hypertension.[11]

For the primary composite end point, all subgroups responded more favorably to losartan than atenolol treatment, although statistical significance was not attained for the 25% RR (95% confidence interval [CI] = 0.56–1.01) in the ISH group. The subgroups also demonstrated that losartan had the most consistent and dramatic impact on stroke, most prominently the 40% reduction in the ISH group and least prominently (21%) in the diabetic group (hazard ratio (HR) = 0.79, 95% CI = 0.55–1.14).

Table 11.1
ARB trials in hypertension and stroke medicine.

Study	Ref	Treatment groups*	Duration (years)	Selected inclusion criteria	Primary end point	End point	RR (95% CI)	p
Losartan Intervention For Endpoint reduction in hypertension (LIFE)	6	• Losartan ± HCTZ • Atenolol ± HCTZ	4.8	• Age 55–80 years • SBP 160–200 and/or DBP 95–115 mmHg • ECG-LVH	Composite of CV death, MI, and stroke	Primary	Adjusted 0.87 (0.77–0.98) favoring losartan	0.021
						CV death	Adjusted 0.89 (0.73–1.07) no difference	0.206
						MI	Adjusted 1.07 (0.88–1.31) no difference	0.491
						Stroke	Adjusted 0.75 (0.63–0.89) favoring losartan	0.001
						NODM†	Adjusted 0.75 (0.63–0.88) favoring losartan	<0.001
Study on COgnition and Prognosis in the Elderly (SCOPE)	40	• Candesartan ± HCTZ • Placebo ± HCTZ	3.7	• Age 70–89 years • SBP 160–179 and/or DBP 90–99 mmHg • Mini-Mental State Examination score ≥24	Composite of CV death, MI, and stroke	Primary	10.9% (−6.0–25.1%) no difference	0.19
						Stroke	23.6% (−0.7–42.1%) borderline significance favoring candesartan	0.056
						CV death, MI	No difference (data not provided in reference)	NS

Study		Years	N	Inclusion criteria	Endpoints			p
Valsartan Antihypertensive Long-term Use Evaluation (VALUE)	• Valsartan • Amlodipine	4.2	15 245	• Age ≥50 years • Untreated SBP 160–210 and DBP <115mmHg, or treated SBP ≤210 and/or DBP ≤115mmHg • High CV risk	Primary cardiac events (sudden cardiac death, fatal MI, death during/following PTCA/CABG, death due to HF, MI on autopsy, new-onset HF requiring hospitalization, non-fatal MI, and emergency revascularization or thrombolytic/fibrinolytic treatment to avoid MI)	NODM	0.75 (no CI reported) trend favoring candesartan	0.09
	42					Primary	1.04 (0.94–1.15) no difference	0.49
						MI	1.19 (1.02–1.38) favoring amlodipine	0.02
						Stroke	1.15 (0.98–1.35) trend favoring amlodipine	0.08
						NODM	0.77 (0.69–0.86) favoring valsartan	<0.0001

Table 11.1
Continued

Study	Ref	Treatment groups*	Duration (years)	n	Selected inclusion criteria	Primary end point	Selected results		
							End point	RR (95% CI)	p
MOrbidity and mortality after Stroke, Eprosartan compared with nitrendipine for Secondary prevention (MOSES)	44	• Eprosartan • Nitrendipine	2.5	1405	• Hypertension requiring treatment • Cerebrovascular event within last 24 months	Composite of total mortality and all CV and cerebrovascular events, including recurrent events†	Primary	0.79 (0.66–0.96) favoring eprosartan	0.014
							CV events	0.75 (0.55–1.02) favoring eprosartan	0.06
							Cerebrovascular events†	0.75 (0.58–0.97) favoring eprosartan	0.03

ARB, angiotensin receptor blocker; CABG, coronary artery bypass graft; ECG-LVH, electrocardiographic left ventricular hypertrophy; HCTZ, hydrochlorothiazide; PTCA, percutaneous transluminal coronary angioplasty; BP, blood pressure; HF, heart failure; CI, confidence interval; CV, cardiovascular; DBP, diastolic blood pressure; MI, myocardial infarction; NODM, new-onset diabetes mellitus; PVD, peripheral vascular disease; Ref, reference; RR, relative risk; SBP, systolic blood pressure.
† NODM is measured in the patients without diabetes at baseline. Consult the referenced literature for numbers of patients at risk of NODM.
* The MOSES trial differs from the LIFE study in that the MOSES population was required to have prior stroke and therefore recurrent strokes were analyzed. Furthermore, the LIFE study only included first events in analyses; whereas MOSES included first and recurrent study events

In both the no CVD and ISH groups, new-onset diabetes was significantly less in the losartan group, paralleling the findings for the entire LIFE cohort. Hospitalizations for angina were consistently non-significantly higher in the losartan groups of the substudies, whereas in the diabetic group fewer patients treated with losartan were hospitalized for heart failure ($p = 0.019$).

The occurrence of sudden death was not significantly different between treatment groups in the overall LIFE cohort.[12] In the subgroup with diabetes, there were 44 occurrences of sudden death, 44% of all cardiovascular deaths. Fourteen of these deaths occurred in the losartan group compared with 30 deaths in the atenolol group ($p = 0.027$). Fewer sudden deaths were observed in the losartan group than in the atenolol group in patients with diabetes and atrial fibrillation (6% vs 13%).[12]

ECG-LVH regression

It had previously been shown that regression of LVH in hypertension related to improved prognosis.[13] By 6 months of treatment, both the Cornell product and Sokolow–Lyon voltage had declined significantly, with statistically greater declines in the losartan group ($p < 0.001$).[14] The difference in the ECG-LVH regression was consistent and statistically significant at $p < 0.001$ over the course of 5 years of treatment. Beginning at 6 months of treatment and continuing throughout, significantly fewer patients in the losartan group had LVH by both criteria ($p < 0.001$ at all measurement intervals). Furthermore, regression lines plotting the change in systolic BP versus the change in either the Cornell product or Sokolow–Lyon voltage demonstrated that for any change in systolic BP, the regression of ECG-LVH was consistently greater for the losartan group.[14]

The Framingham study demonstrated that the odds of having cardiovascular disease were increased in patients who had an increase in serial voltage change on the ECG as opposed to a decrease.[15] Consequently, the greater decrease in ECG-LVH evident in the losartan group may have contributed towards the reduction of events in the composite end point of the LIFE study. Furthermore, previous work has demonstrated that cerebrovascular events are more common in patients with ECG-LVH.[16] The fact that losartan produced a greater regression of LVH with similar BP control provides a possible mechanism to explain the reduced occurrence of stroke that was noted in the overall LIFE cohort and the subsequent subgroup analyses.

Serum uric acid

In the LIFE study, baseline serum uric acid (SUA) was significantly associated with increased cardiovascular risk (HR = 1.024, 95% CI = 1.017–1.032 per 10 μmol/L increase).[17] Losartan attenuated the increase in SUA in comparison with the atenolol (17.0 ± 69.8 vs 44.4 ± 72.5 μmol/L, $p < 0.0001$) over the duration of the study. Furthermore, it was shown that 29% of the reduction in the primary composite end point with losartan could be explained by the difference in SUA over the course of the study ($p = 0.004$).[17] A trend toward an interaction of gender with SUA was not significant; however, the association with time-varying SUA and risk was higher in women ($p < 0.0001$) than in men ($p = 0.0695$). In men, there was a strong relationship of the Framingham risk score (along with degree of LVH, a prespecified adjustment in the risk models), which complicates the interpretation of these results.

The association between cardiovascular risk and SUA is well accepted, but the causality is not. In the LIFE trial, the effect of losartan on the relationship of cardiovascular risk to SUA was more profound in women than in men. The enigma presented by these findings adds further to the controversy surrounding cardiovascular risk and SUA. Nevertheless, the LIFE trial suggests that the unique uric acid-lowering quality of losartan may be an added benefit of this particular ARB.

Urinary albumin excretion

The association of microalbuminuria with 'benign' essential hypertension was first documented in 1974[18] and only later associated with cardiovascular disease and mortality.[19–21] It was also found to be associated with LVH in the LIFE study,[22,23] Losartan was associated with reductions in albuminuria that were 33% and 25% greater than with atenolol (both $p < 0.001$) after the first and second years of study in the 8206 patients who had measurements.[24] Although baseline albuminuria did not clearly identify patients who benefited the most from losartan, one-fifth of the benefits of losartan on the primary composite end point could be statistically accounted for by losartan's greater effect on reducing albuminuria.[24] Thus, the antiproteinuric effects of losartan exerted an apparent protection against cardiovascular outcomes in the LIFE cohort, adding to its known renal protective effect in patients with type 2 diabetes and nephropathy from the results of the Reduction of Endpoints in NIDDM with the Angiotensin II Antagonist Losartan (RENAAL) study.[25]

Characteristics of LVH Determination by ECG

By analyzing the prevalence of LVH by both Cornell product and Sokolow–Lyon voltage against tertiles of BMI, the LIFE study demonstrated that obesity had a greater effect on LVH determination by the Sokolow-Lyon voltage method than the Cornell product method.[26] A progressive increase in the Cornell product was noted as BMI tertile increased, but a progressive decrease in the Sokolow–Lyon voltage was observed.

Further examination of the characteristics of LVH determination by the Cornell product and Sokolow–Lyon voltage was also performed.[27] The Cornell product criterion was satisfied by 65.9% of patients, whereas the Sokolow–Lyon voltage criterion was met by only 23.1% of the sample. Multivariate analysis revealed that the best predictors of LVH by Cornell product were higher BMI, increased age, and female gender. The Sokolow–Lyon voltage was predicted by lower BMI, male gender, and black race.

The presence of albuminuria was also investigated in relation to the ECG-LVH. Baseline albuminuria was independently associated with diabetes, higher BP, older age, serum creatinine, smoking, and ECG-LVH.[22,23] Following 1 year of treatment, the decline in albuminuria was independently associated with regression of ECG-LVH,[28] leading to the conclusion that albuminuria represented generalized vascular damage.

Echocardiography

In 906 patients with measurable echocardiographic mass and baseline ECG measures, 75% had ECG-LVH at screening and at baseline. Because of regression to the mean, 25% did not satisfy ECG criteria for LVH at baseline but did at screening. Those found to satisfy criteria at both time points had increased prevalence of echocardiographic LVH (86% vs 55%, $p < 0.001$).[29] The ECG criteria used to identify patients with LVH indicated a prevalence of >70% by echocardiographic measures of LVH.[30]

In 750 patients who had complete measures of LV dimensions and Doppler filling patterns, correlates were observed.[31] Multiple regression analysis demonstrated that LV mass correlated with isovolumetric relaxation time, but LV mass and geometry were not related to peak early LV filling velocity (E), peak atrial filling velocity (A), or mitral valve E-peak deceleration time. The E/A ratio was independently correlated with isovolumetric relaxation time.

LIFE patients were also compared with groups of 282 employed hypertensive and 366 apparently normal adults to study wall stress and myocardial oxygen demand (measured as a triple product of heart rate, mass, and wall stress).[32] The LIFE subjects (who were heavier and older than the comparison groups) had substantially supranormal wall stresses and increased triple product compared with the other groups when compared by gender. These changes indicate an increased myocardial oxygen demand and predisposition for myocardial ischemia in the LIFE cohort. The main LIFE study and substudies indicated no difference between losartan and atenolol with respect to MI, even though the β-blocking action of atenolol decreased heart rate, a component of the triple product and correlate of myocardial oxygen demand.

Systolic function was also a topic for the echocardiographic substudy.[33] LV mass was the strongest correlate of impaired endocardial shortening and midwall shortening. In patients characterized with eccentric LVH, depressed endocardial shortening was most common, whereas patients with concentric remodeling or hypertrophy demonstrated impaired midwall shortening. It was later demonstrated in blinded treatment analyses that 3 years of antihypertensive therapy improved systolic LV performance, associated with decreases in LV mass, relative wall thickness, and BP and an increase in stroke volume.[34]

In a separate analysis that addressed those patients with ISH vs those with combined hypertension, relative wall thickness was independently associated with ISH, supporting the concept that systolic BP is stronger than diastolic BP as a determinant of end-organ damage.[35]

Because atrial fibrillation has a high association with stroke, correlates of left atrial size were also determined. It was found that 56% of women and 38% of men had enlarged left atria. Left atrial enlargement was found in multiple logistic regression to be related to LVH and eccentric geometry, increased BMI, systolic BP, age, mitral regurgitation, female gender, and atrial fibrillation.[36] Repolarization ECG correlates of ventricular arrhythmias, namely the QT interval and QT dispersion, were found to be significantly related to the LV mass index and LVH.[37]

Atrial fibrillation

The risk of new-onset atrial fibrillation was reduced by 33% ($p < 0.001$), independent of covariates, on losartan- vs atenolol-based therapy,[38] and the risk of cardiovascular events was reduced by about 40% with losartan in patients with new-onset ($p = 0.03$)[38] or established ($p = 0.009$)[39] atrial fibrillation.

Summary

The LIFE study demonstrated that a treatment regimen based on losartan was superior to a regimen based on atenolol in preventing cardiovascular end points in patients with hypertension and LVH, despite similar BP control during 4.8 years of follow-up. These effects were generally observed in the subsets of the LIFE cohort with higher risk, namely patients with ISH and diabetes, but also in patients with no previous clinical history of cardiovascular disease. The most profound treatment effect was on stroke, whereas no significant differences could be demonstrated over the cardioprotective effects of β-blockade with atenolol on MI.

The regression of ECG-LVH was also greater in the group treated with losartan, providing a possible mechanism for its protective action in comparison to atenolol. Additionally, reduction in end points in the losartan group could be related to less of an increase in SUA, to greater reduction of albuminuria, and to greater benefits with regard to atrial fibrillation in the losartan group.

The findings of this study have verified the importance of treatment with losartan in patients with hypertension and ECG-LVH.

SCOPE

The Study on COgnition and Prognosis in the Elderly (SCOPE) followed 4937 patients with a mean age of 76 years old for 3.7 years (see Table 11.1).[40] In addition to assessing the effect of candesartan compared with placebo plus conventional treatment (diuretic) on major cardiovascular events, SCOPE tested the hypothesis that antihypertensive therapy would prevent the decline in cognitive function associated with hypertension.[41] Cognitive function was well maintained in both the candesartan and the control groups.[40] There was a significant risk reduction in the candesartan group for non-fatal stroke (RR = 0.72, $p = 0.04$) and a non-significant trend toward a decreased risk of major cardiovascular events. Both groups had significant BP reductions, but the change in the candesartan group was significantly greater ($p < 0.001$) compared with the control group.[40]

VALUE

Design and execution

The Valsartan Antihypertensive Long-term Use Evaluation (VALUE) trial randomized 15 313 hypertensive patients with high cardiovascular risk into a double-blind comparison of valsartan-with amlodipine-based treatment (see Table 11.1).[42] A total of 15 245 randomized patients were included in the analysis, and 68 patients in 9 centers were excluded because of good clinical practice deficiencies. Only 90 patients (0.6%) were lost to follow-up. The mean duration of exposure to study medication was 3.6 years in both treatment groups. The median daily doses were valsartan 151.7 mg and amlodipine 8.5 mg. As indicated in the 30-month analysis, the majority of patients in both groups were on combination treatment. Fewer patients in the valsartan-based group (27.0%) than in the amlodipine group (35.3%) remained on monotherapy during the course of the study.

Blood pressure control rates in VALUE were among the highest reported for an outcome trial: 56% of patients in the valsartan group and 62% of patients in the amlodipine group reached target blood pressure levels below 140/90 mmHg. These numbers should be viewed in light of the fact that although 92% of patients were treated for hypertension at baseline and many received more than one drug, only 22% had their BP controlled at baseline.

Particularly during the first 6-month treatment adjustment period, the blood pressure-lowering effects of the amlodipine-based regimen in VALUE were more pronounced than those of the valsartan-based regimen. Differences in systolic/diastolic BP were 4.0/2.1 mmHg after 1 month and were reduced to 1.5/1.3 mmHg after 1 year ($p < 0.001$ between groups). Despite these differences, there was no difference in the primary outcome of composite cardiac end points between the valsartan and amlodipine groups.

Outcomes

The primary end point occurred in 10.6% of patients in the valsartan arm and in 10.4% of patients in the amlodipine arm (HR = 1.04, 95% CI = 0.94–1.15, $p = 0.49$). Rates of all-cause death were not different between the groups (HR = 1.04, 95% CI = 0.94–1.14, $p = 0.45$). Of the secondary end points, fatal and non-fatal MI occurred in more patients on valsartan-based therapy (HR = 1.19, 95% CI = 1.02–1.38, $p = 0.02$) although it should be noted that this was due to lower rates of non-fatal events with amlodipine (HR = 1.22, 95% CI = 1.04–1.44, $p = 0.02$) and that the rates of fatal events were not different between the treatment groups (HR = 1.04, 95% CI = 0.74–1.47, $p = 0.81$). There were trends towards fewer heart failure hospitalizations in the valsartan group (HR = 0.89, 95% CI = 0.77–1.03, $p = 0.12$) and more strokes (HR = 1.15, 95% CI = 0.98–1.35, $p = 0.08$). Notably, new-onset diabetes developed in 690 patients on valsartan-based therapy and in 845 patients on amlodipine-based regimens (odds ratio = 0.77, 95% CI = 0.69–0.86, $p < 0.0001$). This is the first demonstration of benefits in the prevention of diabetes with an ARB compared with a metabolically neutral antihypertensive agent.

Tolerability was good in both groups, but the most common adverse event, edema (including peripheral edema), was twice as common in amlodipine-treated patients as in valsartan-treated patients. Hypokalemia was more frequent in the amlodipine group. Although of low frequency, dizziness, headache, and diarrhea were more frequently reported in patients on valsartan-based regimens. Discontinuation rates from adverse events were significantly lower with valsartan-based treatment (13.4% vs 14.5%, $p = 0.045$). It should be noted that the rates of adverse events were somewhat higher than those reported previously for these drugs, almost certainly reflecting the influence of the agents that were added to the primary treatments.

Importance of reaching blood pressure target

Because the aim of VALUE was to achieve control of BP by 6 months, it was assessed whether reaching this goal would affect outcomes for each of the drug groups. HRs for subsequent clinical events in patients with systolic BP <140 mmHg at 6 months were compared with those whose systolic BP was not controlled within each treatment group. Control of BP was a powerful determinant for the primary and secondary end points (except MI), as well as for all-cause death. The differences between the two groups were so minor that the data could be pooled to show the overall role of blood pressure control in optimizing outcomes. These findings provide evidence to validate the target recommendations (140/90 mmHg) in hypertension guidelines from Europe and the USA for this high-risk population.

Importance of blood pressure difference

The early BP differences between treatment groups in VALUE made the overall results difficult to interpret. In an attempt to test the hypothesis in a controlled population, the technique of serial median matching was applied to the dataset at 6 months.[43] Although a post hoc analysis, this method should be considered in plans for new studies, and perhaps even tested in previously reported studies with substantial blood pressure inequalities. The method selected the most median patient (based on systolic BP) within the valsartan group and paired this patient with one from the amlodipine group matched for systolic BP (within 2 mmHg), age, sex, and the presence or absence of previous coronary disease, stroke, and diabetes. The process was repeated until all eligible patients were included. In this way, 5006 comprehensively matched valsartan/amlodipine cohort pairs (a total of 10 012 patients) were created, with a mean systolic BP of 139.9 mmHg in each drug group. The analysis of this patient population, where essentially patients at the high and low extremes of achieved BP were excluded, showed a non-significant trend in favor of valsartan for the combined cardiac end point. The rates of fatal and non-fatal MI, stroke, and mortality were close to identical in both treatment groups. However, admission to hospital for heart failure was significantly ($p = 0.040$) lower with valsartan.

Summary

The results from VALUE underscore that in hypertensive patients at high risk for cardiac events, achieving blood pressure targets is a highly important determinant of outcomes. Most of these patients should be on combination therapies. If BP is controlled, VALUE indicated that valsartan-based therapy is associated with a reduced risk for heart failure hospitalizations, and is otherwise closely similar to amlodipine for other cardiovascular end points. Furthermore, regardless of BP, valsartan-based treatment was associated with a significantly reduced number of cases of new-onset diabetes. These data were obtained with a valsartan dose range of 80–160 mg, which is less than the 160–320 mg now recommended in the USA.

MOSES

The MOrbidity and mortality after Stroke, Eprosartan compared with nitrendipine for Secondary prevention (MOSES) study randomized 1405 high-risk hypertensive patients with stroke during the previous 24 months to a mean of 2.5 years of eprosartan- or nitrendipine-based therapy (see Table 11.1).[44] BP was reduced similarly in both treatment arms, with >75% of patients achieving goal pressures (<140/90 mmHg). The primary end point of all-cause mortality and all cardiovascular events, including recurrent ones, was reduced by 21% ($p = 0.014$) and cerebrovascular events were reduced by 25% ($p = 0.03$) on eprosartan-based therapy.

ONTARGET and TRANSCEND

The ONgoing Telmisartan Alone and in combination with Ramipril Global Endpoint Trial (ONTARGET) is designed to test whether blockade of the AT_1 receptor offers similar benefit to ACE inhibition and whether the combination of angiotensin receptor blockade and ACE inhibition has a greater effect on clinical outcomes than either mechanism alone. ONTARGET is assessing the effect of telmisartan alone, ramipril alone, and their combination on the composite cardiovascular end point of cardiovascular death, MI, stroke, and hospitalization for heart failure in 23 400 patients 55 years old or older at high risk for adverse events but who do not necessarily have hypertension (Table 11.2).[45] The trial, which is expected to last 5.5 years, is

Table 11.2
Ongoing ARB trials in hypertension, prevention, and stroke medicine.

Study	Ref	Treatment groups	Duration (years)	n	Selected inclusion criteria	Primary end point	Comments
ONgoing Telmisartan Alone and in combination with Ramipril Global Endpoint Trial (ONTARGET)	45	• Telmisartan • Ramipril • Telmisartan/ ramipril	5.5	25 620	• Age > 55 years old • Hypertension optional • History of CAD, stroke, PVD, or diabetes mellitus with end-stage organ damage	Composite of CV death, MI, stroke, and hospitalization for HF	Completion expected in 2007
Telmisartan Randomized AssessmeNt Study in aCE iNtolerant subjects with cardiovascular Disease (TRANSCEND)	45	• Telmisartan • Placebo	5.5	5000 projected	Patients screened for ONTARGET who are intolerant of ACE inhibitors	Composite of CV death, MI, stroke, and hospitalization for HF	Completion expected in 2007
Scandinavian Candesartan Acute Stroke Trial (SCAST)	46	• Candesartan • placebo	1.5	2500	• Hypertension (SBP >140 mmHg) • Acute stroke	Mortality and/or dependency	Secondary outcomes: composite CV events
Randomized Olmesartan And Diabetes MicroAlbuminuria Prevention study (ROADMAP)	*	• Olmesartan • Placebo	5.0	4400	• Type 2 diabetes • Hypertension, smoking, obesity, or lipid abnormality • Normoalbuminuria	Development of microalbuminuria	Secondary outcomes: composite CV events, reduced renal function and retinopathy

Abbreviations, see Table 11.1. In addition: CAD, coronary artery disease; PVD, peripheral vascular disease; ACE, angiotensin converting enzyme.
*Information taken from ROADMAP News 2005, No. 1.

also investigating the mechanisms of action of angiotensin II and exploring functional and morphologic consequences of inhibiting the peptide.

Patients screened for ONTARGET who are intolerant of ACE inhibitor therapy are being randomized to a parallel study (Telmisartan Randomized AssessmeNt Study in aCE iNtolerant subjects with cardiovascular Disease [TRANSCEND]) with the same primary end point and an expected enrollment of 5000 patients (see Table 11.2).[45]

SCAST

Scandinavian Candesartan Acute Stroke Trial (SCAST) is designed to investigate the potential benefit of the ARB candesartan vs placebo in patients with acute stroke and concomitant systolic BP >140 mmHg at admission (see Table 11.2).[46] The primary end point is a combination of mortality and dependency, and all cardiovascular events are secondary. Patients are given as much as 16 mg of candesartan over the first 7 days, with a follow-up phase of 180 days. The study needs 2500 randomized patients and an estimated 2 years to complete enrollment.

ROADMAP

Randomized Olmesartan And Diabetes MicroAlbuminuria Prevention study (ROADMAP) compares the ARB olmesartan with placebo on the development of microalbuminuria in 4400 patients with high risk, including hypertensives and diabetics. Cardiovascular end points are secondary.

Perspectives regarding treatment of hypertension

ARBs are exceptionally well tolerated, with side effects that have been similar to placebo control. The main indication for ARBs is the treatment of hypertension. Their BP-lowering abilities have been extensively investigated and appear to be of the same magnitude as other commonly prescribed antihypertensive drugs. Although the ideal antihypertensive combination appears to include low doses of HCTZ, ARBs may, in principle, be combined with any other class of antihypertensive drugs. When combining an ARB with potassium-sparing diuretics, control of electrolytes is recommended. The ARBs should not be used in suspected or known pregnancy, and effects on serum creatinine may be untoward in patients with renal artery stenosis, particularly if the condition is bilateral.

Never before has a class of drugs become so quickly tested in large-outcome studies in hypertension, diabetes, nephropathy, post MI, heart failure, and post stroke. Approximately 100 000 patients have been investigated in prospective, randomized clinical trials with hard end points, and more large trials are ongoing. Some of the trials suggest superior protection against stroke and several show lowered risk for new-onset diabetes. Risk for heart failure may be reduced. There are numerous potential beneficial effects of treating patients with these disorders with ARBs.[47] Recently, some confusion was created regarding risk for MI using ARBs by a review of selected studies.[48] However, a later and updated overview including all the ARB trials[49] indicates that this class of drugs is neutral compared with other drug classes for hypertension in this aspect.

In conclusion ARBs are exceptionally well tolerated and have target-organ protective abilities – a message that patients need to be told. Ongoing clinical trials will also contribute to determining the overall role of ARBs in the treatment of patients with and at high risk for cardiovascular disease.

Summary

The goal of treating hypertensive patients is to prevent target organ damage and cardiovascular complications. Most antihypertensive drugs lower blood pressure effectively and thereby lower cardiovascular risk. The LIFE and SCOPE studies showed that angiotensin II receptor blockers (ARBs) losartan and candesartan were superior to older therapies for lowering risk for stroke and new-onset diabetes. Recently, the MOSES study with eprosartan suggested that ARBs could lower the risk for cardiovascular end points more effectively than calcium channel blockers in stroke survivors. The VALUE trial in high-risk hypertensives, however, showed no significant difference for valsartan compared with amlodipine for lowering cardiovascular risk, but valsartan lowered risk for new-onset diabetes. Ten years have come and gone with the ARBs, with approximately 100 000 patients in clinical trials. The ARB clinical trial program has been one of the most extensive in the history of cardiovascular drug research, and has established the drug class as an attractive choice for most hypertensive patients for primary and secondary cardiovascular protection. Ongoing trials such as ONTARGET, TRANSCEND, SCAST, and ROADMAP will also contribute information regarding the overall role of ARBs in the treatment of patients with and at high risk for cardiovascular disease.

References

1. Volpe M, Ruilope LM, McInnes GT, Waeber B, Weber MA. Angiotensin-II receptor blockers: benefits beyond blood pressure reduction? J Hum Hypertens 2005; 19:331–9.
2. Staessen JA, Wang JG, Thijs L. Cardiovascular prevention and blood pressure reduction: a quantitative overview updated until 1 March 2003. J Hypertens 2003; 21:1055–76.
3. Dahlöf B, Devereux R, deFaire U et al. The Losartan Intervention for Endpoint Reduction (LIFE) in Hypertension Study; rationale, design, and methods. Am J Hypertens 1997; 10: 705–13.
4. Norman JE Jr, Levy D. Improved electrocardiographic detection of echocardiographic left ventricular hypertrophy: results of a correlated data base approach. J Am Coll Cardiol 1995; 26:1022–9.
5. Anderson KM, Wilson PW, Odell PM, Kannel WB. An updated coronary risk profile. A statement for health professionals. Circulation 1991; 83:356–62.
6. Dahlöf B, Devereux RB, Kjeldsen SE et al. Cardiovascular morbidity and mortality in the Losartan Intervention For Endpoint reduction in hypertension study (LIFE): a randomised trial against atenolol. Lancet 2002; 359:995–1003.
7. Lindholm LH, Ibsen H, Borch-Johnsen K et al. Risk of new-onset diabetes in the Losartan Intervention For Endpoint reduction in hypertension study. J Hypertens 2002; 20:1879–86.

8. Kjeldsen SE, Dahlöf B, Devereux RB et al. Effects of losartan on cardiovascular morbidity and mortality in patients with isolated systolic hypertension and left ventricular hypertrophy: a Losartan Intervention For Endpoint reduction (LIFE) substudy. JAMA 2002; 288:1491–8.

9. Devereux RB, Dahlöf B, Kjeldsen SE et al. Effects of losartan or atenolol in hypertensive patients without clinically evident vascular disease: a substudy of the LIFE randomized trial. Ann Intern Med 2003; 139:169–77.

10. Lindholm LH, Ibsen H, Dahlöf B et al. Cardiovascular morbidity and mortality in patients with diabetes in the Losartan Intervention For Endpoint reduction in hypertension study (LIFE): a randomised trial against atenolol. Lancet 2002; 359:1004–10.

11. Kjeldsen SE, Julius S, Hedner T, Hansson L. Stroke is more common than myocardial infarction in hypertension: analysis based on 11 major randomized intervention trials. Blood Press 2001; 10:190–2.

12. Lindholm LH, Dahlöf B, Edelman JM et al. Effect of losartan on sudden cardiac death in people with diabetes: data from the LIFE study. Lancet 2003; 362:619–20.

13. Verdecchia P, Schillaci G, Borgioni C et al. Prognostic significance of serial changes in left ventricular mass in essential hypertension. Circulation 1998; 97:48–54.

14. Okin PM, Devereux RB, Jern S et al. Regression of electrocardiographic left ventricular hypertrophy by losartan versus atenolol: the Losartan Intervention For Endpoint reduction in hypertension (LIFE) study. Circulation 2003; 108:684–90.

15. Levy D, Salomon M, D'Agostino RB, Belanger AJ, Kannel WB. Prognostic implications of baseline electrocardiographic features and their serial changes in subjects with left ventricular hypertrophy. Circulation 1994; 90:1786–93.

16. Verdecchia PM, Porcellati CM, Reboldi G et al. Left ventricular hypertrophy as an independent predictor of acute cerebrovascular events in essential hypertension. Circulation 2001; 104:2039–44.

17. Hoieggen A, Alderman MH, Kjeldsen SE et al. The impact of serum uric acid on cardiovascular outcomes in the LIFE study. Kidney Int 2004; 65:1041–9.

18. Parving HH, Mogensen CE, Jensen HA, Evrin PE. Increased urinary albumin-excretion rate in benign essential hypertension. Lancet 1974; 1:1190–2.

19. Yudkin JS, Forrest RD, Jackson CA. Microalbuminuria as predictor of vascular disease in non-diabetic subjects. Islington Diabetes Survey. Lancet 1988; 2:530–3.

20. Damsgaard EM, Froland A, Jorgensen OD, Mogensen CE. Microalbuminuria as predictor of increased mortality in elderly people. BMJ 1990; 300:297–300.

21. Kuusisto J, Mykkanen L, Pyorala K, Laakso M. Hyperinsulinemic microalbuminuria. A new risk indicator for coronary heart disease. Circulation 1995; 91:831–7.

22. Wachtell K, Olsen MH, Dahlöf B et al. Microalbuminuria in hypertensive patients with electrocardiographic left ventricular hypertrophy: the LIFE study. J Hypertens 2002; 20:405–12.

23. Ibsen H, Olsen MH, Wachtell K et al. Reduction in albuminuria translates to reduction in cardiovascular events in hypertensive patients: losartan intervention for endpoint reduction in hypertension study. Hypertension 2005; 45:198–202.

24. Ibsen H, Wachtell K, Olsen MH et al. Does albuminuria predict cardiovascular outcome on treatment with losartan versus atenolol in hypertension with left ventricular hypertrophy? A LIFE substudy. J Hypertens 2004; 22:1805–11.

25. Brenner BM, Cooper ME, de Zeeuw D et al, RENAAL Study Investigators. Effects of losartan on renal and cardiovascular outcomes in patients with type 2 diabetes and nephropathy. N Engl J Med 2001; 345:861–9.

26. Okin PM, Jern S, Devereux RB, Kjeldsen SE, Dahlöf B; Group FT. Effect of obesity on electrocardiographic left ventricular hypertrophy in hypertensive patients: the Losartan Intervention For Endpoint (LIFE) Reduction in Hypertension Study. Hypertension 2000; 35:13–18.

27. Okin PM, Devereux RB, Jern S et al. Baseline characteristics in relation to electrocardiographic left ventricular hypertrophy in hypertensive patients: the Losartan Intervention For Endpoint Reduction (LIFE) in Hypertension Study. Hypertension 2000; 36:766–73.

28. Olsen MH, Wachtell K, Borch-Johnsen K et al. A blood pressure independent association between glomerular albumin leakage and electrocardiographic left ventricular hypertrophy. The LIFE Study. Losartan Intervention For Endpoint reduction. J Hum Hypertens 2002; 16:591–5.

29. Okin PM, Devereux RB, Jern S et al. Relation of echocardiographic left ventricular mass and hypertrophy to persistent electrocardiographic left ventricular hypertrophy in hypertensive patients: the LIFE Study. Am J Hypertens 2001; 14:775–82.

30. Devereux RB, Bella J, Boman K et al. Echocardiographic left ventricular geometry in hypertensive patients with electrocardiographic left ventricular hypertrophy: The LIFE Study. Blood Press 2001; 10:74–82.

31. Wachtell K, Smith G, Gerdts E et al. Left ventricular filling patterns in patients with systemic hypertension and left ventricular hypertrophy (the LIFE study). Losartan Intervention For Endpoint reduction. Am J Cardiol 2000; 85:466–72.

32. Devereux RB, Roman MJ, Palmieri V et al. Left ventricular wall stresses and wall stress-mass-heart rate products in hypertensive patients with electrocardiographic left ventricular hypertrophy: the LIFE study. Losartan Intervention For Endpoint reduction in hypertension. J Hypertens 2000; 18:1129–38.

33. Wachtell K, Rokkedal J, Bella JN et al. Effect of electrocardiographic left ventricular hypertrophy on left ventricular systolic function in systemic hypertension (The LIFE Study). Losartan Intervention For Endpoint reduction. Am J Cardiol 2001; 87:54–60.

34. Wachtell K, Palmieri V, Olsen MH et al. Change in systolic left ventricular performance after 3 years of antihypertensive treatment: the Losartan Intervention For Endpoint reduction (LIFE) Study. Circulation 2002; 106:227–32.

35. Papademetriou V, Devereux RB, Narayan P et al. Similar effects of isolated systolic and combined hypertension on left ventricular geometry and function: the LIFE Study. Am J Hypertens 2001; 14:768–74.

36. Gerdts E, Oikarinen L, Palmieri V et al. Correlates of left atrial size in hypertensive patients with left ventricular hypertrophy: the Losartan Intervention For Endpoint Reduction in Hypertension (LIFE) Study. Hypertension 2002; 39:739–43.

37. Oikarinen L, Nieminen MS, Viitasalo M et al. Relation of QT interval and QT dispersion to echocardiographic left ventricular hypertrophy and geometric pattern in hypertensive patients. The LIFE study. The Losartan Intervention For Endpoint Reduction. J Hypertens 2001; 19:1883–91.

38. Wachtell K, Lehto M, Gerdts E et al. Angiotensin II receptor blockade reduces new-onset atrial fibrillation and subsequent stroke compared to atenolol: the Losartan Intervention For End Point Reduction in Hypertension (LIFE) study. J Am Coll Cardiol 2005; 45:712–19.

39. Wachtell K, Hornestam B, Lehto M et al. Cardiovascular morbidity and mortality in hypertensive patients with a history of atrial fibrillation: the Losartan Intervention For End Point Reduction in Hypertension (LIFE) study. J Am Coll Cardiol 2005; 45:705–11.

40. Lithell H, Hansson L, Skoog I et al. The Study on Cognition and Prognosis in the Elderly (SCOPE): principal results of a randomized double-blind intervention trial. J Hypertens 2003; 21:875–86.

41. Kilander L, Nyman H, Boberg M, Hansson L, Lithell H. Hypertension is related to cognitive impairment: a 20-year follow-up of 999 men. Hypertension 1998; 31:780–6.

42. Julius S, Kjeldsen SE, Weber M et al. Outcomes in hypertensive patients at high cardiovascular risk treated with regimens based on valsartan or amlodipine: the VALUE randomised trial. Lancet 2004; 363:2022–31.

43. Weber MA, Julius S, Kjeldsen SE et al. Blood pressure dependent and independent effects of antihypertensive treatment on clinical events in the VALUE Trial. Lancet 2004; 363:2049–51.

44. Schrader J, Luders S, Kulschewski A et al. Morbidity and Mortality After Stroke, Eprosartan Compared with Nitrendipine for Secondary Prevention: principal results of a prospective randomized controlled study (MOSES). Stroke 2005; 36:1218–26.

45. Teo K, Yusuf S, Sleight P et al. Rationale, design, and baseline characteristics of 2 large, simple, randomized trials evaluating telmisartan, ramipril, and their combination in high-risk patients: the Ongoing Telmisartan Alone and in Combination with Ramipril Global Endpoint Trial/Telmisartan Randomized Assessment Study in ACE Intolerant Subjects with Cardiovascular Disease (ONTARGET/TRANSCEND) trials. Am Heart J 2004; 148:52–61.

46. U.S. National Institutes of Health Clinicaltrials.gov Protocol Registration System. Scandinavia Candesartan Acute Stroke Trial (SCAST). Available at: http://clinicaltrials.gov/ct/show/NCT0012003. Accessed July 26, 2005.

47. Ruilope LM, Agabiti Rosei E, Bakris GL et al. Angiotensin receptor blockers: therapeutic targets and cardiovascular protection. Blood Press 2005; 14:196–209.

48. Verma S, Strauss M. Angiotensin receptor blockers and myocardial infarction. BMJ 2004; 329:1248–9.

49. McMurray J. Angiotensin receptor blockers and myocardial infarction: analysis of evidence is incomplete and inaccurate. BMJ 2005; 330:1269.

Index

Note – Bold page numbers refer to figures; tables are indicated by italic page numbers.

Printed and bound by CPI Group (UK) Ltd, Croydon, CR0 4YY

23/10/2024

01777708-0005

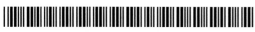